Professional Burnout in Medicine and the Helping Professions

ABOUT THE EDITORS

Dorsey Thomas Wessells, Jr., EdD, is a Licensed Professional Counselor in private practice in Virginia Beach and Newport News, Virginia. In addition to his psychotherapy practice, Dr. Wessells consults with a variety of health professionals, business personnel, police, and educators on stress management and professional burnout. Dr. Wessells has conducted numerous studies on stress and burnout for helping professionals, published a variety of articles, and contributed to numerous books on these subject areas.

Austin H. Kutscher is President of The Foundation of Thanatology, and Professor of Dentistry (in Psychiatry) at the College of Physicians and Surgeons, Columbia University, in New York City. His clinical and teaching activities have focused on psychosocial aspects of life-threatening illness and bereavement; cancer diagnosis, therapy, and management; and pharmacotherapeutics. Dr. Kutscher is the editor of *Loss, Grief & Care*.

Irene B. Seeland, MD, is Assistant Clinical Professor of Psychiatry at New York University Medical Center and Attending Psychiatrist at Goldwater Memorial Hospital. She has been working with terminally ill patients as a liaison psychiatrist for 20 years. Dr. Seeland previously worked for Beth Israel Hospital (Mount Sinai Medical Center) and Columbia Presbyterian Medical Center on the Oncology Unit. She has presented workshops and lectures throughout the United States and Europe on the theme of death and dying.

Florence E. Selder, PhD, RN, is Associate Professor and Urban Research Center Scientist, University of Wisconsin at Milwaukee. She is in private psychotherapy practice at the Midwest Center for Human Services, Milwaukee. Dr. Selder, co-author of *Human and Ethical Issues in the Surgical Care of Patients With Life Threatening Diseases*, has contributed many articles on thanatology and nursing to professional journals.

Daniel J. Cherico, PhD, is Director of Program and Policy for The Foundation of Thanatology and a staff member at Columbia Presbyterian Medical Center. He has lectured, conducted workshops, and participated in interdisciplinary educational programs and seminars concerned with current problems in caregiving for life threatened, terminally ill patients, their family members, and the health care staff.

Elizabeth J. Clark, PhD, is currently an Associate Professor of Health Professions and Assistant to the Dean of the School of Professional Studies at Montclair State College in Upper Montclair, New Jersey. Her specialty areas are social oncology and thanatology, and she has published a variety of articles about these topics. Dr. Clark is the founder of the Social Oncology Network, President of the Sociological Practice Association, as well as a member of the Academy of Certified Social Workers and a Certified Clinical Sociologist.

Professional Burnout in Medicine and the Helping Professions

D. T. Wessells, Jr., Austin H. Kutscher,
Irene B. Seeland, Florence E. Selder,
Daniel J. Cherico, and Elizabeth J. Clark
Editors

Jeanne D. Cole, Publications Manager
Foundation of Thanatology

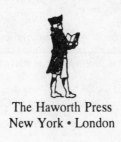

The Haworth Press
New York • London

Professional Burnout in Medicine and the Helping Professions has also been published as *Loss, Grief & Care*, Volume 3, Numbers 1/2 1989.

The Haworth Press, Inc., 12 West 32 Street, New York, NY 10001
EUROSPAN/Haworth, 3 Henrietta Street, London WC2E 8LU England

Library of Congress Cataloging-in-Publication Data

Professional burnout in medicine and the helping professions / D.T. Wessells, Jr. ... [et al.].
    p. cm.
  "Has also been published as Loss, grief & care, volume 3, numbers 1/2 1989 – T.p. verso.
Includes bibliographies.
  ISBN 0-86656-785-2
  1. Medical personnel – Job stress. 2. Allied health personnel – Job stress. 3. Burn-out (Psychology) I. Wessells, D. T.
  [DNLM: 1. Stress, psychological. W1 L0853f v. 3 no. 1/2 / WM 172 P9658]
R609.P76 1988
610.69 – dc19
DNLM/DLC
for Library of Congress
                                                  88-28409
                                                  CIP

Professional Burnout in Medicine and the Helping Professions

CONTENTS

V. COMBATTING BURNOUT

Professional Burnout
in Medicine
and the Helping Professions

Foreword

Alan David Entin

Big Burn. A snow bowl at the top of Mount Snowmass, Colorado. So named after a fire burned down most of the trees near the timberline. An area of tremendous potential, energy, vitality, grandeur and potency burned out, depleted. A hauntingly powerful image engraved in memory.

Burnout is everywhere on the landscape: it is on the physical and emotional landscape and on the interior and exterior landscape. It has become a "catchword" to describe everything and anything in popular and professional jargon, language, literature and culture since Herbert Freudenberger, PhD, originally coined it in the early 1970s. Like expanding concentric circles of rippling waves formed when an object is tossed into the water, this latest book on the subject of burnout enlarges and expands in significant directions the original concept, especially in the innovations in prevention and treatment of professionals most susceptible to its effects. This is its greatest contribution.

It is most appropriate that the book starts with Freudenberger's historical overview of burnout research and current issues in the area. He builds on his previous work on burnout, most notably focusing on the *context* of the burnout situation and, more significantly, the culture, structure and values of the work situation and the impact of the professionals on the culture of the organization. Once again, like the ripples of the water, Freudenberger extends the concept of burnout to include "organizational burnout." It is a recognition that burnout symptoms do not develop in isolation, that there are many reciprocal processes operating in systems to contrib-

---

Alan David Entin, PhD, is a clinical psychologist in independent practice in Richmond, VA, and Fellow, American Psychological Association.

ute to the development and attenuation of burnout. He raises extremely important questions that can occupy the professional lives of many "future burnout researcher(s)."

This book is like a musical score for an overture. The overview, by Freudenberger, introduces the main theme and sets the stage for future evolution and development of the main ideas and concerns of the burnout concept. What follows are developments, elaborations, and variations on the themes introduced in this overview.

The diversity of clinical, research and institutional backgrounds adds to the richness the authors bring to compose the main theme of the book: the development, prevention and treatment of burnout. Although the book is divided into four additional sections, each chapter elaborates and personalizes various aspects of the burnout theme presented in the opening section.

The theme of the section "Burnout and the Professional Care Giver" is on the personal characteristics and attributes of the health care professionals which render them at high risk for burnout. Wessells, a creative "model builder," draws upon the concepts of family systems theory to propose a framework for looking at burnout which every professional can apply to his or her own career. He focuses on reciprocal aspects of over-functioning/under-functioning in helping relationships, developing a sense of responsibility and control of one's own behavior in the definition of job success, and on understanding work as a process, not a product. These are themes that will be echoed throughout the book. Lyall picks up the theme with the message that while "The 'fault' may lie with us . . . so does the solution." It is further elaborated upon by Lynn who suggests that "To ignore all these mundane things is to invite burnout." Combined, these chapters present "simple and basic" ideas that are nonetheless "viable ways to fend off burnout." Stevenson addresses how educators can translate professional priorities into attainable, often short-term, tasks which provide a sense of accomplishment for vulnerable professionals. Keeping the "limbic look" alive, the "glow of the eyes," is the central theme of Regelson's chapter on physician burnout. He offers passionate and eloquent insights into the personality and characteristics of physicians that contribute to their high achievement and vulnerability to burnout. He reiterates Freudenberger's underlying message of the importance of a sense of spirituality. Constructing an "alternative model" of the reality of the health care professional is the model suggested by Rawnsley to minimize burnout.

In the section "Causation Aspects of Burnout" Lyons opens with a provocative essay relating human values and judgments about work experiences. He offers insights into the complex interrelationships between value structures and work expectations. McCarthy looks at the issues involved in altering work habits and lifestyles to deal with the stresses that inevitably lead to burnout. Shifting the emphasis from "a failure to live up to one's ideals" to the necessity of developing a "vision . . . guided by possibilities" is the intriguing insight offered by Selder and Paustian to renew the passion and experience of feeling alive, the "limbic look," and minimize the threat of burnout.

Elaborating on another theme touched upon by Freudenberger, the articles by Sullivan and Weiner each focus on the institutional aspects of burnout and question whether the process is inevitable. They emphasize how most discussions of burnout deal with the way the job affects the individual. However, they offer the needed insights into the other aspects of the process: how the individual affects the job situation.

The "Combatting Burnout" section offers three personal accounts of the interesting processes these diverse health care professionals use for dealing with stressful situations. Weiner applies the teachings of "Self-psychology" to her roles as therapist, consultant, and teacher, finding the commonalities in the "idealization-thermostat" inherent in each role and the hope and optimism afforded by this way of thinking which will enable the worker to develop more effective solutions to avoid burnout. Yarborough discusses his solutions for dealing with his feelings and coping with job stress from the point of view of 40 years in the field of funeral services. He presents a clear motif, which is reiterated in other essays, the need to care for the care giver: "You can't take care of someone else unless you also take very good care of yourself." Also working in a thanatological setting, Clark focuses on process, quality of life, and psychosocial successes as a viable approach to "managing, and perhaps even preventing, the burnout syndrome."

Collectively, these essays broaden the landscape of the concept of burnout. They open new vistas for viewing and understanding this prevalent and potentially devastating phenomenon. By presenting the latest literature, research and techniques for coping with burnout, this volume is a timely and noteworthy addition to the newly emerging field.

Preface

Once several years ago after delivering a paper on professional burnout for medical professionals, I was amazed at the comment of the next presenter as he referenced my remarks. As I recall, this man had a background in hospital administration. His comment addressed my model for describing the ideology and treatment of job stress. He said in effect that my comments certainly pertained to nursing personnel but were not relevant where physicians were concerned. He went on to explain, that physicians were too highly trained to experience job stress much less professional burnout. After this comment, I happened to glance at the moderator of the symposium, a physician, who gave me a knowing smile which I remember to this day.

This experience as much as anything stimulated my interest to help produce a symposium and text that explored stress and burnout issues specifically in the area of medicine and the helping professions. In reading the chapters contributed by a cross section of physicians and helping professionals interested in this topic, I believe we have created a practical hands on book that will aid in the identification and reduction of job stress in this specialized group.

This text achieves what no earlier work has attempted for medicine and the helping professions. First, it offers a thorough understanding of professional burnout. Further, it elaborates on how burnout develops. Through a systems approach, it offers a generic model for the reader to identify job stressors unique to his or her work setting. It enables the reader to explore the cognitive and interpersonal aspects that contribute to job stress and ultimately burnout. Secondly, the text offers an in depth exploration of stress and burnout issues from the perspectives of specific medical and helping profession disciplines. Some disciplines covered are physicians, nurses, social workers, psychotherapists, teachers, consultants, agency and hospital workers, funeral directors and others.

Of particular value is the language of this text. We strove to have these articles readable by the cross section of disciplines covered. Even in the instances of reports on original research, the material is presented in such a manner that one need not be highly versed in statistical, psychological or medical jargon to find this book useful.

D. T. Wessells, Jr.

I. AN OVERVIEW OF BURNOUT

Burnout:
Past, Present, and Future Concerns

Herbert J. Freudenberger

The rapidity with which the term and the concept of burnout have been incorporated into the daily argot of our society is astonishing. During the last five to eight years, burnout has become a buzz word used to convey a great number of personal and social problems.

I brought the concept of burnout to professional and public awareness in 1973 (Freudenberger 1974, 1975). The newness of the field compels our attention to certain practical and theoretical pitfalls that often beset the development and evolution of a new concept (Freudenberger 1983).

First, let us trace the origin of the term and development of the concept. It evolved from work I did within the free clinic movement, an alternative model of general health care established in the 1960s to serve young people who had rejected the "establishment." Over some time, we began to note significant changes in mood, attitude, motivation and personality among the volunteers who were working in the free clinic. These individuals came from a

Herbert J. Freudenberger, PhD, is in independent practice, New York, NY. He is Fellow, American Psychological Association, and author of *Women's Burnout* and *How to Beat the High Cost of Success*.

1

variety of personal and professional backgrounds. Some were parents whose children had run away or were in difficulty; others were people who wanted to help the many "hippy" youngsters who nightly came into our clinic seeking medical, dental, drug and psychological assistance. Other volunteers were young professionals — nurses, dentists, physicians, social workers, counselors, and psychologists — who recognized that a need existed and were there to offer assistance (Freudenberger 1974).

Historically, the concern of those professionals who became involved in the study and wrote of the burnout concept dealt with the personality and clinical aspects of the individual. Cherniss wrote, "we found that many of the new professionals we studied did change during the first year or so of their careers. They lost much of their idealism. They became less trusting and sympathetic toward clients, students or patients" (Cherniss 1980).

Other clinicians observed the many ways that burnout impeded functioning in a large variety of fields. Austin began to speak about the field of social workers. He commented that "the profession of social work services requires a more comprehensive view of the worker as client, with particular reference to job satisfaction and occupational health" (Austin and Jackson 1977).

Belcastro spoke of teacher stress and burnout. He found that "somatic complaints are indeed significant discriminating variables between burned out teachers and teachers who are not burned out" (Belcastro and Gold 1983).

Cynthia Beck, in her study of burnout in teachers of retarded and nonretarded children in a rural environment, found "significant differences in the degree of burnout experienced by three groups of teachers." It is interesting that teachers of mentally retarded students scored significantly lower on symptoms of burnout than did other teachers. One explanation for this might be that these teachers have fewer pupils, have greater use of paraprofessional aides, and may, through a personal selection process, approach their work with "superhuman qualities and abilities" (Beck 1983).

Burgess, in turn, spoke about stress and burnout in the nursing profession. She said stressors had their origin in "patient-care issues, self expectations, interstaff issues and institutional demands" (Burgess 1980).

As time went on, studies and observations were reported on physicians, clergy (Freudenberger 1982), librarians, child care workers (Freudenberger 1977), veterinarians, pharmacists, attorneys, judges, police officers (Freudenberger 1982), dentists (Freudenberger 1986), psychotherapists/psychoanalysts (Freudenberger 1979, 1985), and air-traffic controllers.

The articles and reports were increasingly replete with observations and symptoms of what constitutes burnout. Bramhall and Ezell (1981) suggested that burnout was manifested through some of the following observable symptoms: withdrawal, becoming callous and cynical, making sick jokes, ridiculing the client, becoming mentally exhausted, and suffering from psychosomatic complaints, headaches, backaches, gastrointestinal problems, anxiety, inability to concentrate, and depression.

As time went on, we came to general agreement on what the symptoms of burnout were, but issues were raised about the meaning of the term itself. Some definitions in the literature are vague, contradictory, or overly inclusive. For example, some theorists refer to burnout as a loss of will or as an inability to marshal one's forces. Others imply that burnout is essentially a pervasive mood. The definitions vary; some are precise, some global, some psychological, some behavioral. Some speak of it as a state, some as a process; some refer to the cause, others only to the outcome, but each has contributed to the understanding of this phenomenon.

As Jackson (1982) suggested, "Despite the differences, there are also similarities. . . . There is a general agreement that burnout occurs at an individual level, that it is an internal experience that is usually psychological in nature," and that it is usually perceived by the individual as a negative experience.

Over usage and over extension tend to make a term meaningless. As Maslach (1981) noted, "not only do the definitions of any single stress disorder vary from each other, but similar definitions are sometimes applied to different concepts." This only adds to the confusion. We need to be careful that we do not place so many concepts under burnout that it becomes meaningless. We do need, however, to prevent premature closure in our thinking; that is, we need to avoid becoming inflexible in our thinking, which might serve as a defense against felt anxieties or felt lack of knowledge.

We need to be careful not to exclude those thoughts that do not agree with our preconceived notions or seek to incorporate more than is possible.

Burnout was initially explored and investigated in the health and social services fields. This was because these fields offered a natural habitat for observing how serious the psychological and behavioral impact of burnout is upon those of us who function in the helping professions. Now, we need to encourage sociologists, biologists, economists, political scientists, industrial-organizational engineers, and corporate personnel to assist us in our explorations of the impact of burnout.

In our explorations, we have begun to shift from exclusively clinical observations of how burnout affects an individual. We have begun to use quantitative instruments, such as the Maslach Burnout Inventory (Maslach 1981). This inventory allows us to quantify, measure and compare burnout variables in various occupational groups and settings.

No discussion of burnout is complete without an evaluation of the structure of an organization, an agency, a hospital, a clinic, or an institution. To what degree do the values, the principles, and the leadership of an institution contain variables and factors that may promote burnout in its staff or personnel?

Cherniss (1980) spoke of "the bureaucratic infringement on a professional's autonomy." He addressed the issue of a professional no longer being able to view himself or herself as a free agent, but rather seeing himself or herself as a person whose function was determined by the value system of the institution for which he or she worked. This set of values often could determine his potential adjustment or maladjustment, the consequences of which, in turn, might lead to burnout. Our burnout thinking must shift to understanding what the forces are that make up the gestalt of an organization.

Most, if not all organizations have a culture of their own. The rites, rituals, values and symbols of that organization are determined by the leaders, by history and by the role characteristics attributed to and performed by those who are functioning on the job. James and Jones (1975) suggest that the following variables tend to determine an organizational climate: "The individual autonomy, the degree of structure imposed upon the position, reward orientations, consideration, warmth and support.'' We also need to consider what values our training institutions and universities impart that do not prepare us for what we will find once we enter our professions and work in our chosen fields.

As we continue our exploration of the concept of burnout, we need to assess the impact on an individual of these organizational values. As suggested by Schein (1985), ''the process of culture formation is, in a sense, identical with the process of group formation. The shared patterns of thought, belief, feelings, and values that result from shared experiences are what ultimately end up being called the culture of the group.'' But what if the value system of the institution is diametrically opposed to the values, ethics and competencies of the individual professional? What if the individual professional seeks to live up to the external, organizationally imposed criteria of what constitutes success and achievement, but is unable to do so? Are these conflicting demands not fertile grounds for burnout of the person? The answer is definitely ''Yes!'' But are these points of internal opposition not also fertile grounds for the burnout of an organization? The answer once again is ''Yes!''

We need to begin to think not only of individual burnout, but also of organizational burnout. I believe that we see this phenomenon, on an almost weekly basis, in the corporate world. ''The raiders,'' the investment and venture capitalists of industry, often pluck a fruit, a corporation, off a tree, when it is ready for takeover. Often the takeover is a consequence of outdated machinery, outdated techniques, poor marketing or sales strategies by inept, rigid, autocratic, or dogmatic executive leadership.

Why doesn't this happen in the social services field? To suggest that some agencies ought to be closed because they are no longer relevant or have outlived their original usefulness would be considered inhuman to the population served. I venture to say that we are sometimes less concerned with the population we serve than we are with our own hesitancies to state that the institution needs to undergo significant change in order to continue to exist. If we do not recognize the reality that the function or philosophy of an organization may have burned out, then we will most assuredly not recognize that we are continuing to burn ourselves and our valued colleagues out in order to sustain these outmoded organizations.

Working with many helping professionals and corporate clients, it has become increasingly clear that the externally imposed societal values of achievement, acquisitions of goods, power, monetary compensation and competition were significant precursors to the eventual burnout that exists in our society (Freudenberger 1980, 1981). Therefore, in order to properly ascertain, cope with and change the root causes of burnout requires looking at the values, ethics, and morality of society, the organization, and finally the individual worker within that institution.

WHAT HAS THE FIELD OF BURNOUT CONTRIBUTED TO SOCIETY?

1. We have introduced and emphasized concepts of stress and burnout into the further consciousness of society. Reflect on how many workshops, seminars, and symposia are being conducted and how many articles are written in magazines, newspapers and journals on stress and burnout.

2. We have helped bring attention to the concept of the impaired professional. For years, those of us who attempted to do so were ridiculed or dismissed when we spoke of troubled, depressed, alcoholic or drug-abusing colleagues. At this time, the nursing, dental, medical, legal, psychiatric, pharmaceutical, clergy, and psychological professions have begun to recognize the problems of impairment and have allowed these colleagues to "come out of the closet" to seek treatment.

3. I believe that the philosophies of wellness programs and of holistic health, which are becoming more accepted within the corporate world, were helped by raising the issues of burnout. Corporations have come to recognize, through their Employee Assistance Programs, that it makes good financial sense to assist employees who are in trouble, and to institute programs that will diminish the possibilities of future medical or emotional problems for such employees.

4. As to the helping professions, we are beginning to give up some of our supermen and superwomen images. We are admitting

that our chosen professions are tough, and we are beginning to give voice to the fact that we feel drained, exhausted, depleted, frustrated, sometimes helpless and depressed. We need to acknowledge burnout in order to continue to contribute to and to promote growth in our students, clients, patients, and ourselves.

WHAT NEEDS TO BE ACCOMPLISHED IN THE FUTURE?

1. We need to develop models that will assist us in structuring burnout research, "Models that will provide a basis for variables to study, as researchers, in order to attempt to predict who will burn out" (Perlman and Hartman 1982). We need to develop models which will assist us in identifying the degree to which personal and organizational variables interact.

2. We need to develop other valid instruments to assist in measuring burnout. We need to establish norms, gathered from homogeneous as well as heterogeneous populations, to ascertain similarities and differences.

3. We need to be quite clear as to "what percentage of professionals, in what profession, working in what type of organization burn out, because of secondary or positive gains associated with this" (Perlman and Hartman 1982).

4. We need to ask such questions as: Do life stages play a part in burnout? Why do some individuals cope more successfully than others? We need to take a closer look at burnout differences between men and women. In my studies over the last three years, significant differences, causes, stages, and consequent adaptations emerged for women (Freudenberger 1985).

5. What stress management techniques make the most sense with what kind of groups? How effective is a workshop if we do not also have impact on the stressors that exist within the organization and on its leadership?

6. We will need to be more efficient in the application of organizational development techniques. We need to explore questions within organizations, such as how we can build in strong support networks and flexibility in job functioning, how we can reduce routine dulling and deadness, and how we can offer opportunities for

individual development and reinforce skills for effective stress resolution while we diminish work overload.

7. We will need to reassess the degrees to which "sociopolitical and sociocultural dynamics may be ultimately linked with burnout" (Dressel 1982). If we only think of burnout in social-psychological, administrative, or organizational terms, we may be shortchanging the concept. The future might necessitate our looking conceptually at the social policies from which service professionals, as well as their clients, benefit or lose. If poor legislation is one source of inadequate funding and uncoordinated service systems, then how will this affect the administrator of an agency? Does this not also affect the amount of paperwork that falls on the service provider? The answer is "Yes!" Therefore our future work in burnout needs to approach the individual, the administration and the organization; it also needs to take into account the macro-sociological and political variables that interact in our society, and ultimately have impact on us, the service providers.

Finally, we can not conclude without mentioning prevention. Prevention will be the cornerstone for our work in the future. We need to develop prevention programs in the schools and we need to prevent burnout in our professional training. Too few institutions speak of impairment while too many professionals are impaired.

We also need to incorporate a sense of spirituality in our work. I do not mean institutionalized religion, rather a sense of morality, ethics, shared values and beliefs. Values should help to promote the human good, and help us face frustration, sadness, stress and ultimately death. We need to develop ways and means, like a good relay team, to pass our knowledge of how to prevent burnout on to the next team, so that they will benefit from our errors and not become enmeshed in the same difficulties.

The above are just a few of the exciting areas that I foresee will concern the future burnout researcher.

In conclusion I would like to quote from Saul Alinsky, who in his book *Rules for Radicals* (1971) said, "the organizer, searching with a free and open mind, void of certainty, hating dogma, finds laughter not just a way of maintaining sanity, but also a key to understanding life." I could not agree more.

REFERENCES

Alinsky, S. 1971. *Rules for Radicals*, 74. New York: Random House.

Austin, M.J. and Jackson, E. 1977. "Occupational health and the human services." *Health and Social Work, 2*(1), 93-117.

Beck, C.L. and Gargiulo, R.M. 1983. "Burnout in teachers of retarded and nonretarded children." *Journal of Educational Research, 73*(3), 169-173.

Belcastro, P.A. and Gold, R.S. 1983. "Teacher stress and burnout: Implications for school health personnel." *Journal of School Health, 53*(7), 10-15.

Bramhall, M. and Ezell, S. 1981. "How burned out are you?" *Public Welfare,* 23-27.

Burgess, A.W. 1980. "Stress and burnout." *Carrier Foundation Letter,* 64.

Cherniss, C. 1980. *Professional Burnout in Human Service Organizations.* New York: Praeger Publishers.

Dressel, P.L. 1982. "Professional Burnout: Sociocultural and Sociopolitical Perspective." Georgia State University.

Freudenberger, H.J. 1974. "Staff burnout." *Journal of Social Issues, 30,* 159-165.

Freudenberger, H.J. (Ed.). 1974. *The Free Clinic Handbook, Journal of Social Issues, 30*(1), 1-210.

Freudenberger, H.J. 1975. "The staff burnout syndrome in alternative institutions." *Psychotherapy: Theory, Research and Practice, 12*(1), 73-82.

Freudenberger, H.J. 1977. "Burnout: Occupational hazard of the child care worker." *Child Care Quarterly, 6*(2), 90-100.

Freudenberger, H.J. and Robbins, A. 1979. "The hazards of being a psychoanalyst." *The Psychoanalytic Review, 66*(2), 275-297.

Freudenberger, N.J. 1981. *Burnout: How to Beat the High Cost of Success.* New York: Anchor Press, Doubleday. Reprinted in paperback, New York: Bantam Books.

Freudenberger, H.J. 1982. "Coping with job burnout." *Law and Order, 30*(5), 5-10.

Freudenberger, H.J. 1982. "Rabbinic burnout; Symptoms and prevention." *Central Conference of American Rabbis Yearbook, XC, II,* pp. 44-52. Columbus, Ohio.

Freudenberger, H.J. 1983. "Burnout: Contemporary issues, trends and concerns." In Farber, B.A. (Ed.), *Stress and Burnout in the Human Service Profession,* 23-29. New York: Pergamon Press.

Freudenberger, H.J. 1985. "Impaired clinicians: Coping with burnout." In Keller, P.A. and R.H. L.G. (Eds.), *Innovations in Clinical Practice: A Source Book 3.* Sarasota, Florida: Professional Resource Exchange.

Freudenberger, H.J. and North, G. 1985. *Women's Burnout: How to Spot It, How to Reverse It and How to Prevent It.* New York: Doubleday.

Jackson, S.E. 1982. Burnout: A concept in need of refinement. Unpublished paper presented at the American Psychological Association.

James, L.R. and Jones, A.P. 1975. "Organizational climate: A review of theory and research." *Psychological Bulletin, 30*(1), 1097-1110.

Maslach, C. 1981. "Understanding burnout problems, process and promise." Paper presented at the First National Conference on Burnout, Philadelphia.

Maslach, C. and Jackson, S.E. 1981. *The Maslach Burnout Inventory*. Palo Alto, California: Consulting Psychologists Press.

Perlman, B. and Hartman, E.A. 1982. "Burnout: Summary and future research." *Human Relations, 35*(4), 283-305.

Schein, E.H. 1985. *Organizational Culture and Leadership*. San Francisco: Jossey-Bass.

The Etiology of Job Stress

D. T. Wessells, Jr.

I have had the opportunity to consult with a variety of helping professionals concerning issues of job stress and professional burnout. With a number of helping professionals, I conducted descriptive research studies designed to identify job stressors unique to a specific profession and job stressors common to most professions. Case examples that follow are drawn from studies conducted over the last five years. These examples will be used to explain the ideology of job stress and develop a model to cope with the stress encountered in our professional lives.

A nurse working in an outpatient Muscular Dystrophy clinic reported increasing feelings of distress in specific areas of her work. She was finding it very difficult to telephone parents of children who attended the clinic on an outpatient basis and were found to be in need of inpatient treatment. Her distress occurred in trying to explain the need for inpatient treatment to upset parents (Wessells, 1983).

A minister described a pattern of repeated feelings of frustration and failure over wanting to say no to some of the demands of his parishioners yet being unable to do so. Frequently after engaging a demanding parishioner on the telephone, the minister would make comments to his secretary that elicited her sympathy for his burdensome task (Wessells, 1982a).

A physician treating children with degenerative illnesses de-

D. T. Wessells Jr., EdD, is affiliated with Associates at Hilton/Lynnhaven, 10354 Warwick Boulevard, Newport News, VA 23601.

This paper was originally presented at the symposium *Professional Burnout in Medicine and the Helping Professions*, sponsored by The Foundation of Thanatology, Columbia-Presbyterian Medical Center, Peninsula Hospital, Associates at Hilton, January 16, 17, 18, 1986 in Hampton, VA.

scribed himself as serving as a "family therapist" to parents of the children he treated. In this light, the physician permitted telephone calls from parents, not of an emergency nature, at all hours. The physician was beginning to appreciate how taxing his professional life was becoming (Wessells, 1986).

Each of the cases cited depicts a professional in jeopardy of professional burnout. The term burnout as it relates to people was coined by Herbert Freudenberger. He defines burnout as a state of fatigue or frustration brought about by devotion to a cause, way of life, or relationship that has failed to produce the expected reward. He goes on to describe the process of burnout as serving to deplete oneself; to exhaust one's physical and mental resources; to wear oneself out by excessively striving to reach some unrealistic expectation imposed by oneself or by the values of society (Freudenberger, 1981). To understand the concept of professional burnout, it is necessary to examine both the cognitive and interpersonal factors that predispose one to burnout. Specifically, how do people's beliefs about their professions cause them to place unrealistic expectations on themselves and others? How one defines job success and responsibility will have a significant influence on whether or not realistic expectations are set. Professionals who evaluate professional success in terms of outcome are in more jeopardy than those who do not. The minister mentioned earlier defined success as pleasing his parishioners. A survey he recently conducted revealed a 96% satisfaction rating of his work by his parishioners. The minister was upset over the 4% not pleased. He often felt he failed when he was unable to accommodate a parishioner. He dared never say no to parishioner demands since such a response would surely result in a disappointed parishioner. This professional is in jeopardy of burnout since success as he defines it is determined by the feelings of others over which he has only limited influence. Because of how he defines success he has no choice but to continue to drive himself to perform a task he cannot accomplish.

Similarly, the nurse cited earlier felt responsible for the wellbeing of those placed in her charge. For her, this implied that she was responsible for somehow ameliorating the upset feelings of the parents she was required to contact about the hospitalization of their children. With each telephone call of this nature, her sense of failure increased since, by her own standards, she was not behaving responsibly. Here again, this professional defined professional responsibility to include things she had no control over, i.e., the feelings of others

The example of the physician, like that of the nurse, involves a professional who feels responsible for the care of those in his charge. In the case of dealing with children with degenerative illnesses, the physician frequently felt he had failed since to him arresting the disease process represented success. His efforts to cope with his sense of failure led him to act as "family therapist" to the parents of his patients in an effort to experience the reward of feeling helpful to these parents in crisis. This additional responsibility added to the problem since it failed to alleviate his sense of failure with the patients, required him to attempt to perform services for which he was not trained and created excessive demands on his time. In this example, unrealistic expectations led the professional to assume additional roles that were equally unrealistic given the absence of training to perform as a family therapist.

In each of these examples, the professionals involved defined job success and responsibility unrealistically. Their own definitions of professional responsibility and professional success served to negate whatever valuable services they rendered and left them feeling that they were failing professionally since they could not attain their goals.

A coronary care nurse reported feelings of frustration and stress in her work. Her primary stressor was a relationship she shared with a physician whom she felt seldom responded adequately to the needs of his patients. She was aware, when feeling stressed over this situation, of becoming more involved with her patients and expressing her upset to her nurse colleagues. She was able to see her overinvolvement with her patients as an effort to compensate for the physician's underinvolvement. What these responses served to do was to take the anxiety she experienced in one relationship and transfer it to other relationships. The effects for the nurse of operating in this manner were several. In channeling her anxiety this way, she avoided any possibility of working out a resolution with the physician who caused the stress. Hence each encounter in which these feelings became aroused in the nurse added to the stress level of the ward, since it required her colleagues to either join with her in objection to the physician or defend the physician. Further, her overinvolvement with her patients had potentially communicated to them her lack of confidence in the physician. Such a communication could undermine patient care. Finally, since there was no way the nurse's overinvolvement could compensate for her perception of physician underinvolvement, the nurse frequently left work feeling exhausted and a failure (Wessells, 1982b).

The chief veterinarian of an emergency veterinary clinic owned by a group of regional veterinarians was ready to resign her position due to job stress. She frequently encountered anxious pet owners who brought in critically and terminally ill pets. Being an emergency service, the rates were higher than nonemergency rates. The outcome of services often was the loss of a pet through injury, illness or euthanasia. Pet owners frequently left the clinic feeling upset by pet loss and high fees. When they shared these feelings with their regular veterinarian, the regular veterinarian automatically joined with the upset pet owner. In turn, the regular veterinarian would require the emergency veterinarian to be accountable about the services rendered at the emergency clinic. This pattern left the emergency veterinarian highly frustrated. Not only was she required to function in a stressful clinical environment, she could not look to her superiors, the regular veterinarians, for emotional support and understanding. In these instances, pet owners elected to take their frustrations to a third party, their regular veterinarians, in lieu of working them out with the emergency veterinarian. What this served to do was transfer the anxiety of the owner to the regular veterinarian and in turn reduce the chances of a resolution to the stressful situation between the owner and emergency veterinarian. The emergency veterinarian found herself constantly defensive and anxious over the services she rendered (Wessells, 1985).

A similar pattern can be seen in the case of the minister mentioned earlier. This professional transferred his stress generated by encountering demanding parishioners to his secretary. Expressing his frustration to her, enabled him to continue to overburden himself by complying with parishioner demands. What it failed to do was give him the impetus to work on learning to say no occasionally to parishioners. Further, this pattern set up the secretary to not voice complaints she may have to her boss whom she had come to see as overburdened. Consequently, stress is likely to build in their relationship.

In the examples of the coronary care nurse, the emergency veterinarian, and the minister, the way stress was handled interpersonally contributed to the stressfulness of the work environment. This occurred due to a failure to seek a resolution to the stressful situation in the relationship in which the stress was produced.

The remainder of this paper will be devoted to developing a model to cope with job stress. To accomplish this, we will consider both the cognitive and interpersonal aspects noted above.

Helping professionals place their vocational energy into helping others to improve physically, emotionally, spiritually, etc. There are many variables that contribute to a "successful or unsuccessful" outcome of these efforts, most of which are beyond the influence of the helping professional. Unlike engineers or mechanics who have more influence over work outcome, helping professionals are faced with the proposition of separating their efforts from all of the other influences on the client in order to judge outcome-based success. An alternative to an outcome focus in evaluating job success requires a shift in emphasis from the effects of one's work efforts to the quality of one's work efforts. Specifically, defining job success based on how one applies one's professional skills rather than on the outcome of the application is realistic. We are in control of and responsible for our own behavior on the job. In this regard we can modify how we do our work to improve our skills, thus bringing job success more within our control.

The Muscular Dystrophy nurse may choose to examine how she defines her professional responsibilities. Is she attempting to be responsible for things beyond her control? In the case of feeling responsible for feelings of her patients' parents, the nurse may choose to redefine her role as supportive listener. In this role she can develop communication skills, learn to be empathetic and handle upset parents. In so doing she can begin to judge her success in this task by how well she applies her skills as opposed to whether or not the parents become upset.

From the study on ministers and burnout from which the earlier minister case is extracted, another respondent dealt differently with the struggle to say no to parishioners. He elected to redefine his role in pastoral care. Unlike his colleague who considered himself responsible for pleasing parishioner demands, this minister defined his role in pastoral care as that of referral agent. He would provide direct services to parishioners' needs he felt equipped to handle based on time restraints and skills required. In cases where time was unavailable or needs could be better met by a referral to another professional, the minister acted as referral agent. In developing a good reference list of referral sources, the minister could feel satisfied in most instances of having dealt successfully with parishioner demands, since making good referrals was a realistic job responsibility.

The physician who dealt with children suffering from degenerative illnesses held himself responsible for arresting the disease process. The realism of holding such a belief is questionable even in situations where the disease in question is a curable one. In instances of degenerative illnesses, such a view is totally unrealistic. While this would seem to be readily apparent, Brice and Bergen found similar patterns in a study on coronary care nurses. Their work revealed that nurses on a coronary care unit, being caught up in the tense atmosphere of the ward, began to feel responsible for the life of the patient (Price and Bergen, 1977). Both in their study and in the case of the physician the professionals lost sight of numerous extemporaneous factors that affect the patient in addition to the treatment (i.e., heredity, willingness to follow medical recommendations, stress in the patient's life, progressiveness of the disease, etc.). It is a simple matter to suggest that the physician redefine his responsibilities to focus more on the quality of care and less on arresting the disease. However, qualities of the professional environment may impact on one's ability to maintain a realistic focus on professional success and responsibility.

Work environments that contain a high level of ambient stress are more likely to elicit unrealistic goals from professionals operating in those environments. Therefore, in order to understand and cope with job stress, it is necessary to deal with the interpersonal aspects as well as the cognitive. In organizations, usually stress is generated in response to or in anticipation of response to an interaction with another person. The interaction can be between supervisor and worker, colleagues or worker and client. How these stressful interactions are handled will influence the level of stressfulness in the work environment. Ideally, stress that is generated in a specific interaction between two people should be resolved in that relationship. When person A is stressed by person B and deals with his upset by confiding in person C, then stress is being transmitted into the work environment. Work environments in which stress is so handled can be thought of as work environments with high levels of ambient stress. Management levels of organizations model how stress will be handled throughout the organization.

In the case of the emergency veterinarian, management elected to deal with stress by redirecting it into the work environment. This occurred when the owner veterinarian joined with the pet owner in taking to task the emergency veterinarian. Recommendations were made to the emergency veterinarian not only to redefine her own definition of success in her work, but to call for a meeting with the board of owning veterinarians to institute new procedures. The procedures to be suggested involved redirecting the stress. The emergency veterinarian requested that owners who encountered upset clients recommend the clients deal directly with the emergency service in airing their complaints with the understanding that, should the issue not be resolved, the client had the option to return to the owner veterinarian with the problem. By establishing this procedure, the opportunity was created for the stressful situation to be resolved. Secondarily, it enabled the emergency veterinarian to begin to experience her superiors as supportive.

The minister who used his secretary as the solution for handling his stress cut himself off from developing new methods to deal with demanding parishioners. He would be well served to redefine his professional responsibilities in realistic terms, perhaps as his colleague was able to do. Once this is established, the minister may elect to use his secretary or others for emotional support, so that he can begin to creatively develop ways of setting limits on demands for his time. His modeling this new behavior to his secretary in turn frees her up to deal with issues she may have with her boss in lieu of protecting him from those issues.

Finally, the nurse who reacted negatively to the physician whom she thought provided too little attention to the patients, would be well served to attempt to resolve the issue with the physician. In developing an approach to this problem, she may need the support of her colleagues. However, the distinction must be made between using her colleagues to redirect the stress as opposed to using them to help her develop a creative means of dealing with the physician. The former will serve to heighten ambient stress on the ward, the latter to reduce ambient stress as well as stress for the nurse in question.

To summarize, it is necessary in dealing with job stress and professional burnout to be alert to the cognitive and interpersonal aspects of the work place. A professional would be better served to define success in terms of the quality of the process of his work as opposed to the outcome. The professional need only be responsible for things within his or her control. When stress is generated on the job, the goal for the professional is to work for a resolution in the relationship that generated the stress.

It is often difficult in any given professional organization to begin to use colleagues for support who may share common concerns. It is all too easy to have dialogue about a given job stressor develop into gossip that fails to lead to creative problem solving. For this reason, it may be useful to develop formal support groups, preferably led by a mental health professional, in which the issues addressed earlier can be explored in a supportive atmosphere. Such a group will help participants gain objective insight into their professional belief systems as well as direct the dialogue toward problem solving.

REFERENCES

Freudenberger, H. *Burnout: How to Beat the High Cost of Success.* New York: Bantam Books, 1981.

Price, T. and Bergen, B. The Relationship of Death as a Source of Stress for Nurses on a Coronary Care Unit. *Omega*, 1977, 8, 229-238.

Wessells, D. Professional Burnout: An Issue for Those Treating Muscular Dystrophy Patients. *Psychosocial Aspects of Muscular Dystrophy and Allied Diseases.* Illinois: Charles C Thomas, 1983.

Wessells, D. Pastoral Care and Professional Burnout. In B. O'Connor, D. Cherico, C. Smith Torres, A. Kutscher, J. Goldberg, and K. Maraszko, eds.,

The Pastoral Role in Caring for the Dying and Bereaved. New York: Praeger, 1986.

Wessells, D. Job Stress: An Issue for Community Hospital Personnel Treating Patients with Life-Threatening Diseases. In S. Wolf, A. Kutscher, I. Seeland, D. Cherico, E. Clark, and E. Marcus, eds., *The Community Hospital and Its Expanding Role in Thanatology*. Springfield, IL: Charles C Thomas, 1985.

Wessells, D. Family Psychotherapy Methodology: A Model for Veterinarians and Clinicians. *Pet Loss and Human Emotion*. Iowa: Iowa State University Press, 1984.

II. BURNOUT AND THE PROFESSIONAL CARE GIVER

Burnout in the Professional Care Giver: Does the Phoenix Have to Burn or Why Can't Icarus Stay Aloft?

Robert Lynn

I've never been entirely comfortable with the term burnout, perhaps because I envision a Halley's Comet, or the famed Phoenix, or the greasers on the street revving up their Harleys, flexing glistening biceps covered with tattoos, and swilling beer by the six pack. Burnout is probably a term more misused than properly used. For example, is it proper to say that someone who has never achieved anything has burned out? I'm not referring to elitism; I'm referring to the idea that burnout occurs only in achievers. Achievers do not have to be professionals; they can also be craftsmen, laborers, and assembly line workers who "have had it." In one way or another we have all fashioned wings of feathers and wax and, like Icarus, flown too close to a symbolic sun and then plummeted emotionally. This is burnout.

Robert Lynn, MD, is Staff Psychiatrist, Dutchess County Medical Hygiene Clinic, Poughkeepsie, NY.

I'm not going to attempt to define burnout. What seems more important is the descriptive etiology and teleology. Perhaps this can enable us to recognize the entity early on and "effect some preventive maintenance," as the military say. First, let's look at the protean manifestations of burnout as described quite widely in an already overwhelming body of literature. Variations and gradations of burnout, its signs and symptoms are seen in everyone around us and are never considered anything unusual until we notice a pattern of extremes or exaggerations. We even joke about someone having a psychosomatic headache, or taking a long weekend for mental health purposes, or calling in sick for no good reason. We see it and register it but are loathe to piece it together with other clues to label a co-worker as having burnout, perhaps because of the old rationale, "there but for the grace of God go I."

We next turn to stress. Lengthy discussions about the physiology of stress can be better comprehended if read within some context. The two major categories of stress are exogenous and endogenous. Exogenous stressors can be concrete, subtle, or obvious. Good examples of exogenous stressors might be changes in a nurse's shift, the arbitrary transfer to a different service, lack of office space, heavy case loads, or, in the case of a home hospice worker, the travel time to the patient's home. The endogenous stressors are also an amalgam of the concrete, subtle, and obvious. Mixed in are the intricacies of psychological transference and countertransference. A concrete example is patients who have malignancies which will ultimately limit their lives and profoundly modify the quality of their lives. All the reminders are there: the modifications of the body integrity, the loss of an appendage, alopecia, weight loss, pallor, jaundice. How can we avoid these constant reminders?

Care givers dealing with patients with varying diagnoses of malignancy, whether early stages, stages of active and aggressive therapies, or end stages requiring supportive physical and emotional care, are exposed to incredible endogenous stressors. Doctors, nurses, aides, social workers, and hospice workers confront everything from hopefulness to gloomy despair and, in their day-to-day contact with patient and family, their immersion in the family's joys and sorrows becomes inevitable. However, the hospice worker's additional burden is to have missed completely the earlier phases of rejoicing and hopefulness and to be present only at what we, in western culture, consider the tragedy and suffering of waning vitality and the ebbing of life. The closer you get to the family the more you get caught. Remember Josie's fifth birthday party on the ward (there was not to be a sixth)? She long since ceased wanting a two-wheeler which she knew she could not ride anymore. Remember Mike's love for soccer, a game he'd never return to again, or Lisa's early flair for tennis? An episode I'll never forget was that of a young man who had undergone a forequarter amputation, an intra-scapular for a malignancy. His concern was how, if ever, he could ever wear a sport jacket again. It's an indelible image. The longer you work with patients and families the more you learn of their anxieties and worries, their financial difficulties, work lost, and marital problems. It is indeed the rare care giver who can assume "detached concern" as originally advocated in the training of physicians.

In focusing on the weariness and potential for burnout in care givers, we now have an idea as to its etiology and the external and internal manifestations. I'd like to quote from and recommend an especially brilliant and sensitively insightful paper by Paul Pruyser at the Menninger Foundation (1984):

> Sooner or later, health care professionals who deal with conditions entailing much suffering or pain discover that they have to perform a task for themselves in addition to discharging their helping obligations toward their patients. Prone to becoming overwhelmed by the suffering they see around them and fearful of losing their equilibrium, they must undertake an arduous balancing act. When the pain of the world is no longer an abstract philosophical idea but knocks daily at one's door in concrete self-presentations of suffering individuals, safeguards are needed for the continuity of at least some vital restorative processes, such as undisturbed sleep, access to new energy supplies, and some measure of good cheer. But securing such psychological provisions for oneself is not easy, for the very fact that one feels in dire need of such restorative and equilibrating operations is a sign that one's psychological state has already moved in the other direction, where insomnia, tired-

ness, weariness, brooding and a wistful or mournful mood threaten.

His paper also discussed fusion and identification with the patient and how our professional stance and attitudes should protect us from both pitfalls and, at the same time, allow for controlled and limited empathy for the patient's plight. All of this and learning how to deal with the traps of patient's transference and our counter-transference take an emotional toll on our lives. The person in jeopardy of burning out is not alone in suffering the ill effects (Maslach 1982). "Others are singed by burnout. Recipients of care of services, co-workers, family and friends . . . all these people can testify to the costs that the person's burnout has had for them as well."

Stress generated by work can permeate our private lives. It can affect all those relationships on which we depend for restoration. The costs of burnout are immeasurable from the waste of a fruitful career that took a long time and much effort to establish to the effects on patients or clients, the recipients of the care givers' services. We see the results of ineffectual coping strategies or techniques. Burnout is a progressive and chronic state not visible or detected very early because it usually occurs in those strong, self-assured people who mask their weaknesses well.

Burnout is avoidable and preventable but it takes the effort of both the individual and the institution. We can expect that sensitive and flexible supervisory personnel can modify work schedules, case loads, physical creature comforts, payroll and benefits expenditures. Environmental factors, like the use of a team approach to limit and dilute personal emotional stresses, can be created. It's considered vital to foster an atmosphere where it's safe to feel and express vulnerability. The use of a group like a team group, which meets weekly as a forum for expressing and sharing both happy and sad experiences with co-workers, is effective. At the original hospice, St. Christopher's, outside of London, there is a weekly meeting with the well known psychiatrist, Colin Murray Parks, to discuss patients as well as feelings. This gives individual team members the opportunity to share their vulnerability and to have healthy and constructive feedback from the rest of the team. Jobs can be adjusted and case loads managed to limit direct patient care and mix in teaching, writing, supervision and administrative responsibilities. Breaks in the work period such as coffee and lunch breaks should not be used to catch up on work. Work should not even be discussed. The time should be used more effectively by going out for a walk or by reading a book.

To ignore all these mundane things is to invite burnout, which will lead to a turnover of personnel about every two years, and even more often in some positions. Consider the loss of time, energy, and money in recruiting and training. Also, this two-year period is the critical time in which burnout can cause people to drop out from their fields completely and enter other fields remote from people-oriented services.

Maslach (1982) has spoken of personal attributes useful in strategies for prevention of burnout. The emotional stability of the care giver is extremely important. A recent study of hospice workers looked at whether or not the worker worked full time in addition to doing hospice work, what the person's religious background was, and whether or not a close family member had died of cancer and how recently. The individual who had had trouble in handling losses in his life, reacting with depressions and distancing behaviors or flight from these losses, should not attempt to work them through by working with the terminally ill. Coping skills and the ability to empathize without merging or fusion is vital. Circumspection and introspection, being able to reflect and be in touch with feelings at all times are important. The ability to use a tool like insight meditation can be life-saving.

What can we do in our day-to-day lives to fend off burnout? Consider "decontamination," or, as Maslach has also put it, "decompression" techniques such as listening to music or books on tapes in the car to help in separating from work. Hobbies are also helpful. Many experts recommend active sports and aerobic exercises, jogging, swimming, yoga. Meditation techniques and relaxation techniques have staunch advocates. And, of course, there's nothing quite like a journey to a distant shore to recharge one's batteries. All of these ideas are so simple and basic that we tend to forget them but they are viable ways to fend off burnout. When death comes and whispers to me, "Thy days are ended," let me say to him, "I have lived in love and not in mere time." He will ask,

"Will thy songs remain?" I shall say, "I know not, but this I know, that, often, when I sang, I found my eternity" (Tagore, *Fireflies*).

REFERENCES

Bates, E.M. 1975. "Stress in Hospital Personnel." *Medical Journal Aust.,* 2:765-767.

Freudenberger, H.J. 1975. "The Staff Burnout Syndrome in Alternative Institutions." *Psychotherapy: Theory, Research, and Practice 12*(1):73-82.

Friel, M. and Techen, C. 1982. "Counteracting Burnout for the Hospice Care-Giver," in McConnell: *Burnout in the Nursing Profession.* New York: CV Mosby, pp. 150-159.

Gardner, E.R. and Hall, R.C.W. 1981. "The Professional Stress Syndrome." *Psychosomatics, 22*(8):672-80.

Hall, R.C.W. et al. 1979. "The Professional Burnout Syndrome." *Psychiatric Opinion, 16*(4):12-17.

Klagsbrun, S.C. 1970. "Cancer, Emotions, and Nurses." *Amer. Journal Psychiatry, 126*(9):1237-41.

Lewiston, N.J. et al. 1981. "Measurement of Hypothetical Burnout in Cystic Fibrosis Caregivers." *Acta Paediatr Scand 70*:935-939.

Lief, H.I. and Fox, R. 1963. "Training for 'Detached Concern' in Medical Students," in Lief et al. (eds.): *The Psychological Basis of Medical Practice.* New York: Harper and Row.

Maslach, C. 1982. *Burnout—The Cost of Caring.* Englewood Cliffs, NJ: Prentice-Hall.

Pruyser, P.W. 1984. "Existential Impact of Professional Exposure to Life-Threatening or Terminal Illness." *Bull. of the Menninger Clinic, 48*(4).

Weisman, A.D. 1981. "Understanding the Cancer Patient: The Syndrome of Caregivers' Plight." *Psychiatry, 44*:161-168.

Wilder, J.F. 1981. "Recognizing Burnout in Health Professionals." *Psychosomatics, 22*(8):653-656.

Winer, J.A. and Ferrano, C. 1984. "Residency Training and Emotional Problems of Physicians." *Ill. Med. Journal, 166*(1):23-26.

Wise, T.N. and Berlin, R.M. 1981. "Burnout: Stresses in Consultation-Liaison Psychiatry." *Psychosomatics, 22*(9):744-751.

The Prevention and Treatment of Professional Burnout

Alan Lyall

To paraphrase Shakespeare, "The fault, dear Brutus, is in ourselves" (*Julius Caesar*) — that we are burned out.

There is an attitude problem that we have perpetuated, and still help to foster throughout society and especially in the helping professions, that leads us to be proud of the fact that we strive to meet unrealistic expectations. If one is a professional athlete, the ability to "play with pain" is a dubious asset since players may not be able to deliver the performance normally expected of them. Yet only a game may be lost.

In the health care system the stakes are much higher and the attitude is much dumber. Yet we traditionally put ourselves and our patients at unnecessary risk by trying to accomplish too much, and we are so proud of our exhaustion that we make no serious effort to remedy the situation.

The fearsome image used to justify this attitude is that people will go untreated, or may even die, if we don't "carry on regardless." This is seldom true. Some acceptance of limitations plus some clever planning can usually improve the service to patients and preserve the health of the clinician.

There is a serious misconception at the root of this ongoing, inappropriate behavior, as illustrated in Figure 1. Our experience teaches us that the harder we try the better we do. This is reinforced by parents, teachers, coaches and employers throughout our lives.

Alan Lyall, MD, is Associate Professor of Psychiatry, University of Toronto Medical School. He is also Head of the Outpatient Department and Psychiatrist-in-Charge of Ambulatory Services, Clark Institute of Psychiatry, Toronto, Ontario, Canada.

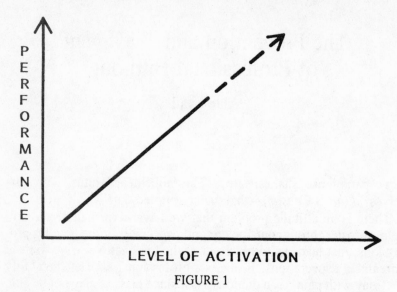

LEVEL OF ACTIVATION

FIGURE 1

The implicit assumption is that such a curve extrapolates ever-upward, forever. When stated this way, however, such a proposition is clearly absurd. Yet, very few people want to consider the implications of what really happens to this performance/activation relationship.

The truth of the matter is that this relationship conforms to an inverted "U" configuration, as in Figure 2.

The implications of the relationship of activation and performance are tremendously important. Up to a point, our performance *does* improve as we become more alert and motivated. But then comes the moment of truth (as the curve plateaus) when such increments no longer augment performance. Subjectively our anxieties are raised and we are usually well programmed to "try even harder." Such a response moves us onto the down slope of the curve and all our incipient fears of failure are fully aroused as we begin, in fact, to fail to meet performance standards.

It is at this point that the subjective experience of stress begins. Up to the apex of the plateau may be what Selye (1976) refers to as eustress and indeed there may be no deleterious effects. However, the concept of eustress can be dangerous since it can be so easily

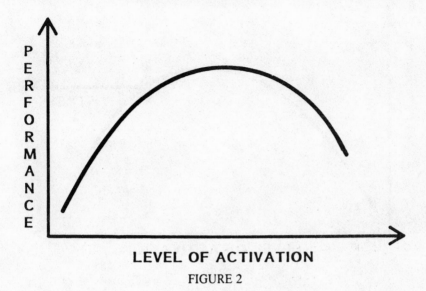

LEVEL OF ACTIVATION

FIGURE 2

misunderstood as to suggest that stress is good for us. Once decompensation begins and we begin to stay "overactivated" it is decidedly unhealthy (Figure 3). We too often rationalize stress as not being so bad; we even come to be proud of our ability to endure it. This is the nature of the attitudinal trap that we concoct for ourselves and often espouse to others.

It is crucial that we train ourselves *not* to increase our pace once symptoms of stress begin to show, but rather to take decisive and immediate steps to do less so that we quickly move back to the healthy side of the curve.

Part of the ethos of being a "pro" is that we strive to meet a challenge, make extra efforts, and don't stop until a task is completed. We are justifiably and properly proud of such an attitude and our abilities to come through. What we lose sight of is the fact that there can be too much of a good thing. Even such a virtuous attitude requires balancing and limiting. It is implicit, rather than explicit, in the Hippocratic Oath that the physician be in good health and be able to provide the best level of care. We require some awareness of how to alter our pace. We must learn how to be unashamed about

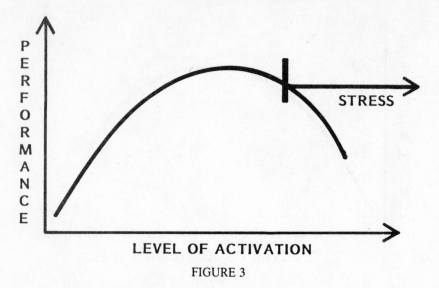

LEVEL OF ACTIVATION

FIGURE 3

acknowledging that we have become stressed. We owe it to our patients and ourselves to remain in a good functioning state.

Too often we fail in the primary task of taking adequate care of ourselves. The anecdotal evidence for this abounds and firmer evidence is accumulating. However, about a decade ago, Mary Vachon and Joy Rogers and I had the opportunity to make direct measurements of the degree of distress among active, front-line professionals in a newly opened Palliative Care Unit of a general hospital (Lyall et al. 1976). We used the short form (30 item) of the Goldberg Health Questionnaire (G.H.Q.) (1972) which is a carefully constructed test with good reliability and validity, originally designed as a screening device to be used in family doctors' offices to select patients who, although clearly not psychotic, might well be sent to a mental health clinic. The cut-off score that suggested that a referral might be appropriate was four.

Amongst the staff of the P.C.U., mostly nurses, we found a score of 9.4. This was double the score found in another newly opened unit of the same hospital, and more than double the score Goldberg suggested was necessary for referral. In a small sub-group who soon left the P.C.U. the average score was 17.

What is important is that these scores were generated by care givers who continued to treat their patients each day. It is at once a tribute to the determination typically found among a professional staff and an indication of how demanding and unrealistic our professions can be. The fact that these scores eventually decreased to more acceptable levels (yet remained close to an average of 4) does not negate how much we often expect of ourselves and of each other.

Any time expectations exceed our ability to perform, we experience stress. We are the chief culprits in defining unrealistic expectations. People are still drawn to the helping professions out of a sense of altruism. When the tasks that need to be done, or could be done, are without limit, the temptation to keep increasing the workload and the pace is virtually irresistible. It becomes a seductive source of personal satisfaction that we can do so much, and most of us carry on until we pay the price.

Learning to slacken the pace and put down some of the load is one of the most difficult things to learn, and many of us never do. There is still too much admiration for those who work excessively long days, neglect personal relationships, and gamble with their health.

Of course, expectations are set not only by ourselves. Group norms gradually emerge in any work setting and our competitive tendencies lead us to try to keep pace with the swiftest. Too often the swiftest are driven by some personal inner demons, so that the whole group constantly accelerates until the wheels start to come off. It is in such a setting, where burnout is becoming common, that patients are often mistreated, not usually in terms of technical mistakes, but rather at the level of neglect of their human needs.

Furthermore, organizations properly set tasks for those within them, and it is very difficult to set realistic expectations for others. It is in the nature of organizations to keep asking for better performance, but it is the individual's personal responsibility to be aware of the organization's excessive demands and to keep the pace reasonable in order to protect him or herself. Lack of a clear statement from the individual on this matter ultimately lets the whole system down. Pace should be an honourable topic of general discussion and negotiation. In the health care professions, we have a responsibility to educate those we serve about the expectations we can reasonably meet.

The "fault" may lie with us, but so does the solution, and learning to alter pace is the key.

REFERENCES

Goldberg, D.P. (1972) *The Detection of Psychiatric Illness by Questionnaire.* Institute of Psychiatry, Maudsley Monographs #21, London: Oxford University.

Lyall, W.A.L., Rogers, J. and Vachon, M.L.S. (1976) "Professional Stress in the Care of the Dying." Presented at the International Seminar on Terminal Care, Montreal.

Selye, H. (1976) *Stress in Health and Disease*. Boston: Butterworths.

Shakespeare, W. *Julius Caesar.*

Professional Burnout in Medicine and the Helping Professions

Robert G. Stevenson

STUDENTS, STRESS, AND BURNOUT

As has been the case in many professions, burnout among educators, both teachers and counselors, is a growing problem. This phenomenon has been attributed to the inability of educators to meet the increasing demands placed upon them and to the growing disparity between their high professional goals and the educators' actual accomplishments, which may fall short of these ideals. Professionals, who were once caring and dedicated, seem suddenly to be merely "going through the motions," devoid of any real emotional commitment to their students.

NEW ROLES/HIGH GOALS

Educators are often assigned new (and unfamiliar) roles with no clear set of behaviors or approaches. They are told to pursue high goals when it is clear that the reality will fall short of the targeted goals. They then find themselves concentrating on the unattained goals rather than on what they may have already accomplished. Faced with new job requirements, new roles to play and new decisions to make, some have decided to stop attempting to adapt to the ever changing and expanding needs of their profession and are content merely to cope with things on a day-to-day basis.

Now we see that even high school students are adopting this pat-

Robert G. Stevenson, EdD, is Co-Chair, Columbia University Seminar on Death. He is Instructor of Death Education Programs at River Dell High School, Oradell, NJ, Bergen Community College, and Fairleigh Dickinson University, NJ.

tern of short-term "coping" while seeking to avoid the pressure from the demand of long-term goals. Two principal methods were developed to help these teachers and students, and it has been found that they represent principles which can be of help to those in fields outside of education, including the medical professions. These include (1) helping the individual to concentrate on living in the present and (2) taking on a new job.

STUDENT BURNOUT

Students operate on a continuum that ranges between helplessness and omnipotence. Their "happiness" is not necessarily based on a realistic view of the world. It has been found that depressed people often have a more realistic view of the world. High school students are confronted with the demands of school, dating, family pressures and college applications at the same time that they are trying to deal with their own biochemical changes, emerging sexuality, self-criticism and demands for increased independence. As has long been true, many adolescents can respond in a positive way to all of these pressures. However, in response to this feeling of pressure, a growing number of adolescents are engaging in self-destructive behaviors like substance abuse or even suicide.

The expectations of success held by students, and those expectations placed on them by family, peers and society, have reached such high levels that reality is almost guaranteed to fall short of the mark they have set. On some abstract level, one might say they had a good life, but they do not see it that way. They feel they are faced with so much pressure that they become unable to differentiate between short- and long-term goals, and, in some cases, become unable to make any decisions at all. Jim's case can illustrate this situation.

Jim was a high school senior who had taken a high-to-average ability and used consistent hard work to maintain a "B" average in honors classes while lettering in three varsity sports. One afternoon, I met Jim walking up and down the hall with a distant look in his eye. I asked him why he was not at practice and he replied that he didn't know. As we talked, he spoke of the many pressures he felt. His parents wanted him to attend an Ivy League college where he thought he might not have the ability to handle the work; his college applications were all overdue; and he had gotten so far behind in two courses that he might fail and not graduate. He had papers to write, clothes to pick up at the cleaners, and even shoes to get soled (since his toes were coming through the ones he was wearing). In addition, he was a twin whose brother had died when they were quite young and he felt that he had to "succeed for two."

Jim had been engaging in polyphasic performance, doing several things at once, for so long that it had become a way of life. He had reached a point where the pressure was more than he believed he could handle. Another young person might have decided to end it all with a suicide attempt. Jim took the "safer" route of deciding not to make any more decisions. This final decision not to decide, while it may have averted any decisions regarding possible self-destruction, also rendered him unable to make any decisions about the most routine day-to-day matters.

The first step in working with Jim was to help him begin to function on a daily basis. He was asked to begin to list all of the things he felt had to do, both short-term and long-term. Then the list was arranged in order of priority and schedules were constructed for the next day. As Jim saw the list of jobs grow smaller each day, he began to feel that he could exercise some control over his life again. The next step was family counseling for Jim and his parents to discuss their expectations for Jim's future.

The key step in Jim's dealing with his "burnout" was the realization that only a limited number of goals could be reached in the short term, and that others would have to be postponed until the proper groundwork could be laid. Jim became more selective regarding the jobs toward which he directed his energy and was able to tackle problems one at a time, in the order dictated by *his* priorities. He derived satisfaction from and reduced his anxiety about the future by directing his attention to the present moment.

In restructuring his priorities, Jim used a variation of an ancient Zen koan about a man and a tiger as a guide. A Zen master would present a novice with this story: A man was walking in a wood when he saw a tiger coming after him. He ran as fast as he could but he arrived at the edge of a cliff with the tiger close behind. Rather than be ripped to pieces he leaped over the edge and grabbed hold of a limb that was protruding from the face of the cliff. He looked up and saw that he could not go back, for the tiger was waiting above and as he looked down he saw two more hungry tigers waiting for him to fall. He then looked at the cliff and saw that the branch was coming loose from the cliff. He also saw a wild strawberry plant growing from a crack near the branch. What did he do?

Jim interpreted this story in a way that saw the tigers below as the problems of the future (long-term tasks) and the tiger on the cliff as the problems of the past (his loss of a twin). He could not go back and at present could do little about the future, but he could still use the present moment. He decided to "eat the strawberry" and it was delicious. We cannot live in the past and there are no guarantees of future happiness, but we can try to take full advantage of each present moment.

Since that time, the same method used to help Jim has been used effectively with staff members who feel overwhelmed. They construct their job list, set priorities and try to use each moment to reach the goals which they feel have the greatest priorities.

STAFF BURNOUT

Staff members in a school system have additional constraints which do not apply to students. They face increased responsibilities as the role of the school in the community expands. When the entire educational structure is indicted for shortcomings in some areas, they feel powerless to respond. Those who have spent some time in education look at current literature about teachers and find that they are considered either the "poorest students" who seem to be the only ones willing to enter the profession, or they are the "poorest teachers" who remained when the really talented people left to pursue other careers. This places a teacher in the position of choosing an identity as a "new" incapable teacher, or an "old" incompetent one! Finally, if the teacher still has any illusions about his/her ability to make decisions which will really have an impact on students, he or she will look at the morass which investigative reports say that modern education has become and try to live with the guilt caused by the feeling that, "My decisions helped cause this!"

All of this can be overwhelming to many educators. If their decisions have produced poor results, they stop making any; their initiative disappears. They do the minimum possible and take no work home. They seek to separate their jobs from their home life not because they no longer care about their students, but because they do care and cannot face continued frustration. Educators report sleep disorders and increased feelings of stress as they seek to do less.

Even positive statements from students may not help the situation. Students who see teachers as "problem solvers" place on them the very type of pressure they may be trying to escape. The educator may pull back in anger as if to say, "Don't do that to me!"

Those educators caught in this dilemma are told that they look tired. They rest, and sometimes feel better physically, but the emotional strain is unrelieved. Rather than a rest, it has been found that an effective way of dealing with the educators' negative feedback loop is to allow the teachers or counselors to take on new jobs.

New jobs provide a break from routine, but avoid the guilt which sometimes accompanies inactivity. New jobs should be time limited and have a specific goal. They may or may not deal with people. There must be a method of reaching closure at the end of the tasks (publications of results, verbal or media presentations of findings, implementing a specific change in procedures, to mention a few possibilities). Teacher sabbaticals have performed this function in the past, but financial constraints have caused many systems to stop this traditional practice without fully understanding what the impact of the decision would have on the school staff. To expand alternative jobs for older staff members can actually be more cost effective than eliminating this release time when one considers the renewed energy, optimism and positive results staff members may bring back to their classrooms from such a "limited" job.

These educators are trying to reverse the growing pattern of withdrawal from a profession that had once been a major part of their lives. Successful interventions in cases of student burnout suggested some methods of dealing effectively with staff burnout as well. These methods have proven useful to counselors and teachers (who must increasingly act as counselors) and may also be of value to those in the fields of medicine and the helping professions.

IMPLICATIONS FOR A MEDICAL STAFF

What can medical professionals learn from the experiences of teachers and students? They have high goals (the saving of life) which reality often places out of reach. Demands on their resources are expanding while staff and finances are shrinking. As technology expands, they are being asked to make more and more decisions, each of which could mean life or death for someone in their care, and an increasingly litigious society waits to extract a high price for any "error."

The two prescriptions for educators can be easily applied to those in the medical profession. An individual can construct (or, if needed, be helped to construct) a set of professional priorities. These can then be translated into specific daily goals which can focus on the use being made of the present rather than concentrating on abstract goals which may never be attained. There must also be an opportunity for medical professionals to step aside from their regular routine to tackle a different, short-term task which can provide closure and a sense of accomplishment. Together these two programs may help even medical professionals to use the present to taste the wild strawberries in their lives.

Physician "Burnout"

William Regelson

"Midlife crisis," "burnout," "ennui," and "depression" face many of us when the work challenge is no longer balanced by internal satisfactions, with or without the economic or social need to continue with what we have been doing for most of our lives. This is not a problem related solely to medical practice, since "burnout" has been described as a factor in 45 percent of corporate workers (Golembiewski 1985).

"Burnout" may become a more dramatic problem for society as our life expectancy increases. Within the next few decades, medical research can provide us with the increased opportunity for a healthier life which could reach the absolute limit of 110-120 years. If we can expect 30-40 more years of healthy life, what are we going to do with that added time when sociobiologically we already have problems within a 75-year median life span? Furthermore, if this problem exists in the prestigious, intellectually and economically envied profession of medicine, what echoes of dissatisfaction, ennui and restless frustration exist among those less privileged than we?

Is the shorter life expectancy in the Soviet Union, related to alcoholism, reflected by "burnout" in large segments of their society? Do we have other words for defining the problem when we deal with the socioeconomic and medical problems of poverty stricken people?

In essence, "burnout" reflects dissatisfaction with the workplace, domestic situation and social or political state. Physician "burnout" can be seen as a microcosmic but relatively benign man-

William Regelson, MD, is Professor of Medicine (Oncology), Medical College of Virginia, Richmond, VA.

ifestation of those wider states of dissatisfactions in other socioeconomic groups that can lead to wife beating, drug abuse, child abuse, divorce, racial persecution, suicide, riot, and revolution. While we confine this discussion to physician "burnout," it is a universal plague related to the motivation toward pleasure or endorphin-mediated satisfactions we glean from the workplace and from our personal lives. At one extreme, burnout forces us to change our jobs or living circumstances; at another, it triggers a death wish. We lose the equivalent of an entire medical school graduating class each year in physician suicides (Victoroff 1985), which represents the extreme negative expression of "burnout." We need to anticipate pleasureful events, and we need to maintain hope for the future in order to avoid the depression and despair that can lead to suicide. In workplace terms, we have to be able to gain satisfaction from what we do. We have to be able to turn occupational effort into social or economic values that can provide us with the satisfaction that sustains our motivation.

Medicine, although changing, is still largely a cottage industry of self-motivated practitioners, and the problem of physician, as distinct from corporate, "burnout" is largely an individual problem unrelated to direct managerial practice although bureaucratic demands add to our burden and managerial controls complicate many of our lives as the practice of medicine as a healing art becomes secondary to the corporate or socialized structure.

Those of us in medical practice have made our work the prime focus of our existence, giving recreation and alternative interests much lower priority than other professions do. Those in medicine who defy the stereotypes and maintain a primary interest outside their profession, in the arts, athletics, science or social life, are not common. The identifiable skills that provide our income are the focus of our lives and, for most of us, the focus of our free time.

Upon reaching middle age, we awaken one day confronted by the possibility that we will share the fate of our patients or our parents, and this leads to a need to reappraise our lives. It dawns on us that our omnipotence is illusory and that our medical practice, which demands sympathy, concern, and technical judgment, is too much for us to bear as the major focus of our existence, especially when we are also distracted by petty irritants on many levels. We may still manage to empathize with our patients, but if spouse, child, or parent complains about his or her own lot, we lose our ability to sympathize. Irritability, ennui, sleeplessness, and fatigue may indicate that depression has become manifest and "burnout" is at hand.

Our self-image as physicians is based on the satisfaction we achieve in delivering our professional skills to our patients and patient response to our efforts reinforces our value. The response of our colleagues to our professional identity in terms or referrals, reciprocal involvement or appreciation (i.e., hospital committee and medical society activity) also enhances our self-image and/or income. Suddenly, time catches up with us; the kids have left or completed school; the mortgage has grown small; our parents are ill or dead; a colleague has died or another has had triple bypass surgery. These are compounded by the loss of spontaneity and the decline of an honest enthusiasm for the tennis, golf or jogging that are the socially accepted ways of renewing energy. Man survives by purging the conscious awareness of death and debility from his mind. Our patients and family suffer the debilities of aging, but "perhaps it will pass us by."

Gabbard (1985) has reviewed "the role of compulsiveness in the normal physician." He feels physicians are almost all compulsive, characterized by a "restricted ability to express warm and tender emotions, perfectionism, insistence that others submit to one's way of doing things, excessive devotion to work and productivity to the exclusion of pleasure and the value of interpersonal relations." Gabbard feels that medicine attracts this kind of personality, but, as an academic, in my experience, these personality traits are not apparent in the early freshman and sophomore years of medical school, during the basic science baptism of fire. True, the compulsion to survive academically with competition for grades is a direct heritage of the pre-med contest, but most students have that "limbic look" in the beginning of the medical school experience. The "limbic look" can be identified in the characteristic glow of the eyes, a specific alertness which is the primitive brainstem directly inherited from our feral ancestors where the adrenaline or endorphin reactions equip us for fight, flight, curiosity and the pleasure of existence.

When our eyes and ears are attuned to every nuance of our environment, we are operating at the limbic level. We gaze at our world with the eyes of a three-year old, taking it all in and making new knowledge and experience an integral part of us. The "limbic look" highlights a zest for life and an intense awareness of the world around us. Where does it go? In my experience, there is no doubt that the "look" disappears when "burnout" catches up with us, and, for most medical students, it diminishes with the arrogance and fatigue of the clinical years. Despite this, there are occasional revivals; we fall in love, buy a new car, climb a mountain, get a hole-in-one, take a trip to a foreign country, get elected or appointed to a position of power, or become students again. When we eliminate the hackneyed, the repetitive, the same old sights and sounds, the same smells and people, the world can reverberate once more in our bodies and brains as we encompass new experiences as positive forces and reaffirmations of life. Unfortunately for many of us, when "burnout" develops, the habits of the past and the fears of venturing into the unknown prevent us from coping with the need for change. Fear of change inhibits the revival of the limbus as a transducer for reinterpreting the world as an exciting place.

An excellent personal account of the problems of "burnout" in physicians, entitled *Healing The Wounds*, was recently written by David Hilfiker (1985). The problem for Hilfiker occurred early in his career and he related it to the nature of the practice of medicine itself. I will take the liberty of quoting from his biographical work which so ably explains aspects of the motivational and emotional responses we face in medicine.

> American doctors, whether rural family practitioners or high-tech surgeons, face expectations from their patients, from their own profession, and from the society at large that are utterly unrealistic on a day-to-day basis. They are asked to be Renaissance men and women in an age when that is no longer possible; they are expected to be ultimate healers, technological wizards, total authorities . . . Such expectations add to a rising tide of suspicions of and accusations directed at doctors and medicine, as well as a growing feeling of uncertainty among doctors themselves about the nature of doctoring and of medicine in our society. No wonder that—despite her

prestige, her salary, her power—the physician today is a wounded healer. Who could live up to such a world of expectations without either crumpling or hiding behind the masks of omniscience and omnipotence?

Like many practicing physicians, I entered medicine out of a desire to be of service to people. Whatever other motives I may have had, my root ambition was to help, to respond to others' needs. What I failed to realize, however, was that the very nature of my work as a doctor would push me continually into the position of limiting the help I would give, or ignoring the needs of others . . .

The emotionally healthy life requires a balance, a certain rhythm for moving back and forth between crisis and routine. As a physician, though, I rode continuous roller coasters, both outer and inner; there was simply no occasion to digest what had happened, to think about it, integrate it into my life history. The only way I found to cope was to harden myself to it, to shield myself from it . . .

The blessing and the curse of medicine is that we physicians are privileged to share the most intense moments of life with our patients: birth, death, fear, sorrow, anxiety, disability, healing, joy. These moments are shared without the usual social barriers; thus, we are privy to the deepest of humanity's experiences. But with this privilege comes the burden of availability, of openness to the needs revealed at those intense times. Not surprisingly, I could not sustain the degree of openness required to go from deepest need to deepest need, and consequently I found myself refusing the very service that a major part of me was committed to giving.

Mistakes seem different for doctors . . .

Some mistakes are purely technical; most involve a failure of judgment. Perhaps the worst kind involve what another physician has described to me as "a failure of will." She was referring to those situations in which a doctor knows the right thing to do but doesn't do it because he is distracted, or pressured, or exhausted.

Although I made these sorts of decisions quite routinely for seven years, the cumulative emotional impact was severe. The underlying irrationality of the judgments gnawed at me; the life-and-death importance of my actions kept me awake at night; and the guilt and depression of never really knowing whether I had acted properly wore away at me; for I knew I was being forced into decisions that only God should make.

Paradoxically, as I did my best to manipulate patients into conforming to the needs of an efficiently run office, it was I who became the object, the machine . . . I measured myself at the end of the day by what I had produced. I hung on to my authority and power, since they seemed integral to my work. I certainly recognized the limited power of money to satisfy me, since my income level had become emotionally important to me, money was an important value. Patients' diseases and my services became commodities that were bought and sold at a price.

Perhaps the religious concept of idolatry will be helpful in understanding what was happening to me.

I find Hilfiker's testimony particularly touching because of his search for perfection and concern for humanity. His current personal solution is a nonremunerative search for service as the guide to his own needs. He works in a nonprofit, independent clinic servicing the poor and homeless. He says,

If we are to begin to regain our balance, we must recognize that inherent in the work of doctoring is the concept of servanthood. This is ultimately a mystery; we will always be at odds with ourselves and our world unless we accept the mantle of servanthood along with the role of healer. Finally, each of these beginnings will drastically alter the economics of medicine. Money is the linchpin. Physician incomes must be brought more into line with those of our patients and co-workers.

I view Hilfiker's concern for "idolatry" against the background of my own research and practice in medical oncology in an academic setting. Medical school grantsmanship and research as avenues toward power have led to the appearance of an arrogant new breed of managerial authority whose emphasis is on the control and corporate manipulation of physicians and patients divorced from the humanistic concerns of caring for the ill. While I feel that medicine separated from monetary goals can be of value, I feel that Hilfiker's transfer to a new community of "servanthood" will be only one temporary step in his own search for satisfaction. In private practice, the problems can be compounded by money and greed; in academic life, problems come from power and control. For this reason, I feel that "burnout" still exists as a problem in Israel and Sweden, where income from medical practice is not the predominant motivational factor, although it would be of interest to see if "burnout" exists to the same extent in socialized medical communities. Although we equate money with power, they are not synonymous in situations where political power is the predominant force that governs "burnout." We live in a managerial society. For most of us, it is the ethical values and responsiveness to our needs of management that govern the quality of our lives and have ultimate control of burnout.

While Hilfiker ably discusses some of the important contradictions in medical practice that lead to dissatisfaction, there are other problems, some of which are new and others that have always been part of the medical scene.

1. Economics. Medicine is ceasing to be a "cottage industry." The industrial revolution is here, and health manpower organizations (HMOs), preferred provider organizations (PPOs), corporate medicine, price controls, increased malpractice insurance premiums, bureaucracy, and a growing number of competitive physicians are making it more difficult to practice medicine as a self-contained fraternity of mutual self-interest. After thinking we've made it, we are faced by new groups seeking to control us and making it more difficult for us to earn a living with our egos intact. "Burnout" will be determined by managerial controls governing job satisfaction such as are now evident in the industrial or business workplace.

2. Jealousy, Professional Competition and Power. For years, in academic medicine, I felt that I had a homophobic problem in that I couldn't develop intimate contacts and levels of friendship with male colleagues. As a male, I gave it Freudian connotation and felt that it related to some deep fear of homosexuals. Circumstances led me to leave the medical school environment where I met lawyers, journalists, artists, and even other physicians, far removed from the

medicine practiced in my own backyard, and, suddenly, I realized that it wasn't an intrinsic fear of male companionship that I felt, but the subconscious competitive hostility that exists in academia and is also present in nonacademic practice.

Many doctors have problems of jealousy and competitive fear, whether we admit it or not. We are constantly competing with our colleagues, even in unrelated specialties. If our colleagues are perceived as too successful, we may become jealous or critical of them. One of society's great ills is intellectual jealousy compounded by competition for patients and money. (In academia — add grants and lab space!)

When the "burnout" years approach, these competitive feelings can be more difficult to suppress, particularly if success does not mirror expectations and authority figures, jealous of the capabilities of their colleagues, seek to impose controls to satisfy their own needs. When "burnout" occurs, fighting for a group of patients to prove your intellectual and economic self-worth is suddenly not worth it and going fishing, made possible by a good retirement plan, seems to be considerably more rewarding.

As Gabbard (1985) discussed, we are frequently confronted by colleagues whose life-style requires an "insistence that others submit to one's way of doing things." These individuals thrive by removing threats to their control and destroying competition through innuendo or naked power. For the power broker, this delays his own "burnout" by forcing the retirement of others. It is the external, murderous equivalent to the concept that suicide is frustrated murder directed inward. Forcing others to "burn out" produces a feeling of satisfaction that protects the power wielder from his own dissatisfaction with life.

3. Our Public Image. Once patients loved us and hung onto our every word. Now they want second opinions, informed consent, death with dignity and will check us out in the newspaper health columns or magazines. Ann Landers gets a Lasker Award and malpractice insurance costs make practice in some regions economically impossible.

4. Technologic Displacement and Rotational Responsibility. Increasingly, computers and technicians are replacing our judgmental

skills, and medicine, as an art, is giving way to improved technologies and depersonalized intensive care units.

We are not as needed, and our training in the supportive role as humanistic Oslerian "old clinicians" gets lost because of busy and complex practices. Alternatively, in institutional or group practice settings, our humanistic concerns have been diluted with clinical duties dominated by rotational responsibility and lack of commitment to individual patients. It is easier for us, in group or academic practice, to rotate patient care on an assignment basis.

5. Lack of Recognition. The younger clients don't admire us; the hospital administrators or academic chairmen see us as disposable service units and revenue producers who can be manipulated; lawyers see us as malpractice opportunities, and our patients no longer care that we worked so hard and that we are dedicated healers who came out of prestigious medical schools and residency training programs. No longer "high priests," we are trade union candidates who need to join Local 1199 or the Teamsters' Union to survive!

6. Domestic. Finally, our wives and families may not really care if we drink or smoke too much and our kids are too busy with their own careers. Grandparenting and parenting, as sociobiologic loving experiences, play a vital but limited role. "Burnout" may occur before this aspect of balance to life's satisfactions has established itself. Increasingly true with nuclear families, this is also not strictly speaking a medical problem, but an age-related event.

All the preceding conditions contribute to that moment when one last patient or domestic complaint will drive you to the brink! The clichés to solve the problem have all been enumerated: vacation, hobby, learning a new specialized skill, building a new body, finding a new sexual or economic partner, joining a group, joining the army, becoming politically or religiously active, dabbling in stocks and real estate. "Burnout" leads to retirement when the financial capacities are present, but professional or personal rebirth is of no avail unless the "limbic look" is sought.

"Burnout" leads to suicide when anhedonia, the absence of pleasure as a psychologic or physiologic event, limits the alternatives. One should anticipate pleasure in work, just as one has to experience or fantasize pleasure in love, physical or intellectual activity. One has to have a dream, a vision, in order to survive. We have to find that drug-free experience that will make the endorphins flow. Pleasurable events can come from our personal life-styles or our patient experiences if we can find the time to let our humanistic concerns surface or if we can allow ourselves to be involved with research for other transcendental creative efforts. In summary, we need experiences larger than ourselves. We need religion or a renewed belief in our magical power as healers to provide a focus for our importance to our patients.

Victoroff (1985), in his commentary in the *JAMA*, "My Dear Colleague: Are you considering suicide?" states,

> Elements of your personality, which promised success in medicine early in your education — aggressiveness, ambition, competitiveness, individuality, intellectual avidity, compulsive goal orientation — have prejudiced you to low tolerance to frustration and failure. You have generated an egotistical self-image and expect to be successful and competent in everything. When your resourcefulness, inventiveness, and hours and hours of sustained effort fail, you cannot accept the collapse of idealized expectations. Denial is your universal, nonchemical, addictive defense. You deny fatigue, illness, mood swings, self-doubt, tension under pressure, and your drive for professional prestige and material reward at the expense of those you love.

"Burnout" will come to all of us if we live long enough without seeking to be sensitive to and aware of those around us who would be supportive, loving individuals. This is explained in the myth of Narcissus: As commonly interpreted, Narcissus, drowning in his reflection in the pond, is drowning in the conceit of his own ego image. What the myth really says is that man should not exist solely reflected in his own image, but survives best reflected in the eyes of others. This calls for an effort to make ourselves consciously aware of our value to others and to the world.

Like a medical student imbued with new knowledge, you have to feel you can contribute to the world which honors or is aware of your existence. You exist not because habit and income justify it, but because you are important to others and that enhances your self-worth and reinforces your capacity to experience pleasure.

Your power as a physician can be restored or maintained if you find interest and excitement in the individuality of your patients and your colleagues beyond the confines of your technique. You must be in touch with feelings that provide self-motivation and group involvement. Alternatively, you have to find a setting, another group or an individual who will help support your self-worth. In addition, curiosity, a search for diversity, contact with youth or colleagues in a noncompetitive setting, and a vacation from your patients or current environment is the way to keep the "limbic look" alive. Symbolically, the snake renewing its skin is a metaphor for the possibility, and for most of us, the necessity, of donning the radiant new colors of the renewal process.

REFERENCES

Gabbardo, G.O. 1985. "The role of compulsiveness in the normal physician." *JAMA 254:*2926-2929.
Golembiewski, R. 1985. *Corporate Commentary*.
Hilfiker, P. 1985. *Healing the wounds: A physician looks at his work*. Pantheon.
Victoroff, U.M. 1985. *"My Dear Colleague: Are you considering suicide?"* *JAMA 254*:3462-3466.

Minimizing Professional Burnout: Caring for the Care Givers

Marilyn M. Rawnsley

To be committed to caring for the terminally ill is to risk personal and professional complacency. Persons who are facing the inevitability of death communicate a perspective different from those who are active citizens in the world of ordinary living. Beliefs and attitudes taken for granted in a predictably routine life are called into question by those for whom customary behavior has been disrupted or obliterated by the capricious demands of a life-occluding illness. Care givers hold primary membership in the world of ordinary living; accordingly, the education of health professionals includes socialization in the values of the profession—values that incorporate the myths and mores of society. Care givers enter the professional arena as emissaries of the prevailing culture, a culture from which the terminally ill, assigned a less favorable social status, have been disenfranchised. The dissonance between the lived experience of care givers and terminally ill patients may explain the phenomenon called "professional burnout." Constructs of alternate realities and energy fields are presented here in a model that promotes understanding of professional burnout and suggests strategies for reducing its impact on the practicing professional.

The signs and symptoms of burnout have been described in the literature by authors such as Freudenberger (1980), Maslach (1982), and others. Although fatigue, frustration, negative self-concept and loss of interest in clients consistently characterize the syndrome, speculations vary regarding the factors that precipitate its onset. Two assumptions, the first derived from the writings of Freuden-

Marilyn M. Rawnsley, DNSc, RN, is Visiting Professor, Department of Nursing Education, Teachers College, Columbia University, New York, NY.

berger, and the second from the work of Maslach, are the bases on which I have developed the thesis of this essay. The first assumption is that burnout "is a depletion of energy experienced by those professionals when they felt overwhelmed by others' problems" (Freudenberger 1980, p. 90). The second assumption is that burnout is a type of job stress that "arises from the social interaction between helper and recipient" (Maslach 1982, p. 3).

If a client population's needs or problems are generally perceived by the care giver to be beyond his personal and professional resources, then the probability of burnout is greatly increased. The relationship between available resources and perceived needs and the variables or characteristics of the helper, the patient, and the environment are presented in a model for discussion and analysis in Figure 1. The model is designed to provide a basis for developing hypotheses for research and proposing strategies for practice that can be useful for minimizing the deleterious effects of burnout on care givers, clients, and organizations. If, as postulated, professional burnout is a multidimensional phenomenon involving several individual and environmental variables in a complex interactive process, then focusing on a particular client population in order to examine the conditions under which the interactive process occurs seems warranted. The scope of this essay is limited to an explanation of professional burnout in care givers who work with the terminally ill.

DISCUSSION OF THE VARIABLES

Societal beliefs and attitudes shape the content in which personal and professional values are formed. These societal biases determine which professions are considered essential and they also affect the behaviors of the members of a given profession through their influence on education, licensure, and practice. Contemporary social views on death and dying infiltrate the goals and priorities of organizations that provide care for persons with life-threatening or terminal illness. In a series of classic essays, Aries (1974) critically discussed the evolution of modern attitudes toward death and dying. Aries remarked on an attitudinal change towards acknowledging the reality of death—first motivated to protect the dying person and,

FIGURE 1

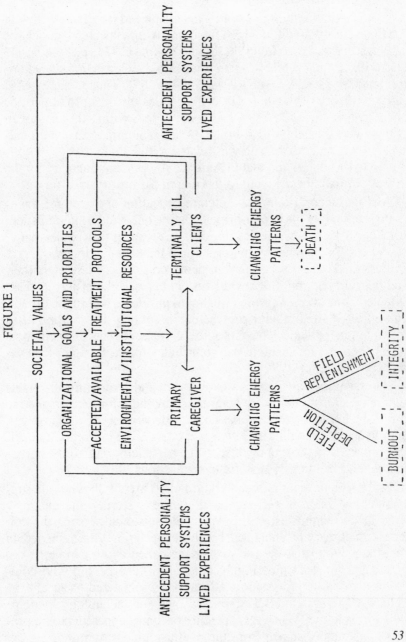

later, to spare the dying person. This misplaced concern created an artificial environment in which the dying were expected "to behave in ways that do not offend the living" (Aries 1974, p. 86-87). He stated that "an acceptable death is a death which can be accepted or tolerated by the survivors" (Aries 1974, p. 89). Thus, acknowledging the finality of death as our common destiny was prohibited, or at least, considered to be in bad taste. Dying within the American culture was particularly complex. Aries maintained that the challenge to the reality of death was related to threats to the social obligation to be happy, and that in America it was compounded "by the search for happiness linked to the search for profit" (p. 100).

Ambiguity contributes to the communication of mixed messages in institutional goals and priorities. On the one hand, quality patient care is promoted as the institution's mission; on the other hand, sound fiscal management policies direct the actual delivery of care. Professionals are assured that in-depth concern for clients is their rightful purpose, but the reward system benefits the efficient, task-oriented employee. Accepted treatment protocols within the organization have a life of their own whether or not they are appropriate to the individual client. A technological culture, such as exists in most of our health care institutions, contributes to an illusion of power and control (Aries 1974).

The resources available to care givers and terminally ill clients within these institutions are determined by the priorities assigned to profit, technology, and compassionate concern for the terminally ill and their professional care givers. Of course, the impact of a death-denying society profoundly affects the perspectives of all the participants, and insidiously distorts their reactions.

Professionals generally enter into the care of those with life-threatening diseases sufficiently inured to suffering and death by their ideals, enthusiasm, altruism, and their own personal health. These qualities are enhanced by the expectation, strengthened in their education, that the rite of passage called dying can be, if not eradicated, at least indefinitely postponed. The person who completes a rigorous professional education is socialized to accept the values of the system. But despite science and technology, patients do suffer and die. When this actuality becomes apparent, some professionals gain distance from the disillusionment by moving away from the direct care giver role and thus avoiding burnout. But some care givers, perhaps because of personality style, perhaps because of limited choices, intensify their involvement in the care of clients for whom death is a highly probable outcome.

The coexistence of different constructions of reality may explain the differences, even the apparent contradictions, that exist in interpretations of experience. Alternate realities were considered by LeShan and Margeneau (1982) to be ways in which persons organized their total experience of the world under particular conditions. Methods for gaining information about these lived experiences included asking the individual directly and observing and analyzing the assumptions or rules that serve as parameters of the reality construction being investigated. LeShan and Margeneau provided a guide for assessing the validity of a given construction of reality:

1. "it must help (you) attain the goals recognized to be valid in that state, or answer the questions defined by its rules as real questions;
2. it must be internally consistent;
3. it must be . . . a state of consciousness that human beings can use and in which, if only briefly, they can continue to function and survive." (LeShan and Margeneau 1982, p. 13)

In this way, the authenticity of alternate realities was distinguished from solipsism, the self-centered view of the world that disregards the reality experienced by others (Wolf 1981, p. 183). Instead, it acknowledged the creativity of consciousness in shaping reality for the individual so that persons who assigned different meanings or sensitivities or who experienced objectively agreed upon events differently can be said to occupy parallel universes. That is to say, their consciousness has shaped alternate constructions of reality (Wolf 1981, pp. 211-225).

Clinical observations and literary accounts of the lived experience of persons who are terminally ill contain recurring themes that can be said to constitute an alternate construction of reality from that of the altruistic, enthusiastic care giver. The patient lives the pain and discomfort of treatments, the hope and discouragement of remissions and relapses, the anxieties of abandonment and dissolution, and the disappointment in the limits of science and technology. The health care professional is at first a bystander. There is no shared agreement on the meaning of the experience. But if a care giver continues to be open to understanding the experience of the patients, communication evolves and energy is exchanged (Rawnsley 1977, pp. 114-116). Judgments are suspended and patterns of reality are shared. The care giver moves between alternate realities.

Repeated experiences of shared realities are intense and exciting. But the patients die, and the energy invested in them is not completely restored. If the lived experiences of the professional who is moving between alternate realities are not communicated to persons who can provide energy replenishment in the form of appreciation and support, then the signs and symptoms of burnout, or energy depletion, begin to appear.

Although it is likely that intervention on global levels of the model, such as societal values, would produce the most dramatic changes, it is also likely that modifications on more concrete operational levels of the system are more readily accomplished. I have had success in working at the level of institutional resources as a process consultant with nursing and social work personnel who care for the terminally ill. The manifest purpose of retaining the services of a consultant outside the institution was to decrease costly professional turnover in outpatient and inpatient oncology staff. The consultant was primarily interested in promoting compassionate care of the terminally ill. Keeping costly turnover to a minimum and promoting compassionate care were not mutually exclusive goals; it was demonstrated that they were complementary. The consultant, who selected the staff as the focus of concern, acted as an intermediary between parallel universes, allowing the care givers to share their lived experience with the patients, reducing the felt dissonance between the alternate realities and replenishing depleted energy through support and guidance. Costly staff turnover and absenteeism decreased and individualized quality patient care was more consistently apparent. Some professionals eventually decided to leave the units for other areas or for more education. But these decisions appeared to be shaped by personal and professional growth motives rather than by the debilitating effects of burnout.

Full explication of the model of reality and its implications for minimizing burnout in professionals has not been possible within the limits of this essay. Likewise, implications for empirical investigation of the relationships of the constructs are the subject for another paper. A quote from the authors of the *Looking Glass Universe* brings appropriate closure to these ideas: "At best we communicate an insight, at worst, an illusion" (Briggs and Peat 1984, p. 103). The verdict is left to those scholars and professionals who will examine the usefulness of the model in suggesting research that can promote our understanding of professional burnout, and in developing strategies that can reduce its incidence in health care professionals.

REFERENCES

Aries, P. 1974. *Western Attitudes Toward Death*. Baltimore: Johns Hopkins University Press

Briggs, J. and Peat, F. D. 1984. *Looking Glass Universe*. New York: Simon & Schuster

Freudenberger, H. with Richelson, G. 1980. *Burn-Out: The High Cost of High Achievement*. New York: Anchor Press, Doubleday & Co.

LeShan, L. and Margeneau, H. 1982. *Einstein's Space and Van Gogh's Sky. Physical Reality and Beyond*. New York: Macmillan

Maslach, C. 1982. *Burnout: The Cost of Caring*. New York: Prentice-Hall

Rawnsley, M. 1977. The Perception of the Speed of Time and the Process of Dying. Doctoral dissertation: Boston University

Wolf, F. 1981. *Taking the Quantum Leap*. San Francisco: Harper & Row

III. CAUSATION ASPECTS OF BURNOUT

A Moral Theory of Burnout: The Evaluation of Work

Richard G. Lyons

As a teenager I regarded working as both liberating and an avenue for recognition. I became more independent and was accorded a measure of prestige. I was satisfied with all those early jobs whether delivering newspapers or working as a clerk. I was satisfied with work not because the jobs were intrinsically satisfying but simply because I began to feel more like an adult. My adult colleagues were harder to please. They complained and invented ingenious ways to make the work day seem shorter. They celebrated their completion of the week. Yet, despite their mixed evaluation of work, they were not burnt out. They had few of the burnout symptoms of exhaustion, low self-esteem, a cynical attitude toward customers, and disappointments over the realities of making a living (McConnell 1982; Edelwich 1980). They were not disappointed since they had a fine grasp of the world of work and how work met some of their needs. They did not invest years in professional train-

Richard G. Lyons, PhD, Professor of Philosophy, University of Lowell School of Nursing, Lowell, MA.

ing to be crushed by the cruel realities of work. Nevertheless, they had some poor job experiences.

My point in this essay is to show that certain job experiences are more important in explaining burnout and work alienation than others. First, I will summarize a recent study on work attitudes which describes six fundamental work experiences. Second, I will argue that these experiences respond to two quite different value orientations. Third, I will suggest that work not only has psychological and historical dimensions but also a fundamental political orientation.

Let me begin with a brief summary of a comprehensive survey of work attitudes conducted by the University of Michigan and the U.S. Department of Labor (Quinn and Stains 1979). The survey charted job experiences of professional and nonprofessional workers to determine how they evaluated their work. The initial survey was conducted in 1969 and was followed by two additional surveys in 1973 and 1977 to see if any trends could be discerned. The study used a factor analysis to establish six dimensions of work experience evaluations: (1) job comfort, which measured such factors as the physical surroundings and hours one needed to work; (2) challenge, which was concerned with the intrinsic rewards of the job; (3) pay, which measured compensation, security, and fringe benefits; (4) relationships to colleagues, which reflected how friendly and interesting the people were with whom one worked; (5) the availability of resources to do the job well; and (6) promotability, which focused on the fairness and opportunity for promotions. Given these standards, Americans dislike their jobs and their dissatisfaction is growing, said Quinn and Stains, and "much of the work in the country is being done under conditions that are unnecessarily onerous, harmful, inconvenient and inefficient" (p. 286).

The demographic data is alarming: men are slightly more dissatisfied with work than women; blacks have more distaste for their jobs than whites; and people under thirty dislike their jobs significantly more than other people. The number of years of schooling no longer serve as a predictor of job satisfaction. With the exception of people with graduate degrees, there is no correlation between years of schooling and job satisfaction. People with high school diplomas are as dissatisfied with working as college graduates. Nevertheless, people without a high school education register more dissatisfaction than people with diplomas. The warning we should be giving children in high school is: if you do not graduate you will have more dissatisfaction than if you finish high school.

Age is a fair predictor of job evaluation. If you exclude people in their twenties, the older you get the less dissatisfied you become with your work. In fact, there is some evidence suggesting that people over 65 have little job satisfaction. Professional and technical job holders, also, enjoy little job satisfaction, which has not changed in the years from 1969 to 1977.

Why do most people experience meaningless work? Two explanations were dismissed by the survey. The first is that too much weight was given to groups who have been characteristically dissatisfied with work. The data does not support this explanation since the decline in job satisfaction affects virtually all subgroups of employment. The second explanation is that the objective qualities and working conditions have decreased. Yet fringe benefits have increased, job accidents and illness have decreased, and workers have increased control over their hours. The slight decrease in wages from 1973 to 1977 explains the decrease in satisfaction with pay but does not explain worker dissatisfaction with other aspects of work.

Another explanation is that people have more ambitious criteria for evaluating work, but the survey does not show any evidence to support or dismiss this explanation. However, this explanation deserves attention since it suggests that job evaluation may be subjective and determined by historical forces. For example, the criteria for a satisfying job during the American Depression in the thirties could have been quite modest: does the job pay a living wage? Older workers, born prior to the Depression, may have had lower work expectations, which could account for their current, more positive, view of work. This example suggests that one's assessment of work cannot be separated from other aspects of living.

Questions about work hinge on broader questions. One third of married workers reported that work interfered with family life, particularly for mothers with young children. Questions about the quality of work may be answered within the context of the quality of life itself. Work evaluation must be seen within a context far broader than employment. Work, in other words, is closely connected with the aspirations and values which govern our lives.

Let me now turn to the issue of life values and how these values have impact on the way we judge working. Frederick Herzberg (1966), the noted industrial psychologist, devised a good model to describe the relationship between human values and our working lives. According to Herzberg, we have two distinct sets of values. The first he calls maintenance or hygiene values. They seek to avoid pain and even death and are directly related to scarcity. The need for food, safety, shelter, clothing, and other conditions for human survival dominate life under conditions of scarcity and danger. When we have met these threats to survival, he suggests a second set of values should be cultivated. Yet, he observes, people are dominated by hygiene values. Clothing, housing, cars, and food consumption continue to play a significant part in our lives well after we have avoided scarcity. Ironically, we find people willing to engage in meaningless work to acquire more of these items. The modern preoccupation with money and material goods, Herzberg argues, reflects only one aspect of personality — namely pain avoidance, whether psychological, like safety, or physical, like hunger.

Survival allows people to nourish a second level of values, that is, psychological growth (Herzberg 1966). Growth has a cognitive as well as an emotional dimension. Cognitively we have a need to have new information and to relate this information to what we believe, creating new patterns and relationships. We must also have the emotional and intellectual stamina to be effective under ambiguous situations where new information and relationships must be nourished by calculated guesses. We must be creative within insecurity. Finally, we must develop a sense of identity which we are willing to defend against the pressures to conform. This implies that social bribes like money, title, awards, and other symbols of success are not substitutes for human growth. The absence of the hygiene factors makes for pain while the absence of growth factors makes for unhappiness. Conversely, the ability to secure the necessities of life creates the conditions for maximum health in which the person is both free of pain and working to his or her intellectual and emotional potentialities.

Herzberg also conducted a study to determine the perceived factors that made work meaningful and unalienating. Working, like living, can be divided into two categories, pain avoidance and growth. What facets of work help us avoid pain? His study suggested that the hygiene factor, or pain avoiders, located in our jobs included the physical working environment, overall company policy toward workers, supervision, relationships with peers, and salary. When some of these factors were absent, the worker experienced job dissatisfaction. One would have thought that if these factors were eliminated or improved, job satisfaction would become evident. His ingenious and creative study suggested a different conclusion: when the hygiene factors at work improved, the long-term effect was not job satisfaction but no job dissatisfaction. When we are not *unhappy* with our jobs we are not necessarily *happy* with our jobs either. For instance, if a person is dissatisfied with his or her salary and the company raises the pay scale, the long-term result is not worker satisfaction. The reason, according to his analysis, is that salary and the other minimum standards satisfy our need to survive and maintain ourselves but not our personality development as spelled out in intellectual and emotional terms. Employers become confused when salary and other minimum factors are improved but workers continue to complain. Their complaints, however, revolve around issues like boring routines and lack of novelty.

People maintain that work, like life, must allow for personal growth. Consequently, our jobs must provide us with an opportunity for achievement and accomplishments, recognition for our work, responsibility to see that our tasks are accomplished, promotion, personal identity, and a challenge to our abilities. These characteristics of work will fill our need to grow psychologically. The reader will notice that work as the means to avoid pain and to provide food, shelter, and the other necessities of life is given a modern context. For example, our relationship with our peers is included as part of the minimum standards. However, the Michigan Survey assumes that all of the categories are equally important in measuring job evaluation. Yet half the categories measure dissatisfaction, that is, salary, job comfort, and relationship with colleagues, while the other half measure satisfaction, that is, challenge, availability of resources, and promotability. One would hope that those aspects of the job which satisfy would outweigh those which do not, especially since salaries and job comfort rate fairly high among the people surveyed.

How would Herzberg's analysis help explain burnout in the help-ing professions? The helping professional may be governed by the factors promoting satisfaction rather than those promoting dissatis-faction. Thus the cure for burnout is quite different if professionals who experience the erosion of such factors as recognition and re-sponsibility. Ironically, if professionals are motivated by factors of dissatisfaction when all other conditions, such as salary, are met, then they are simply neurotic but they are not burnt out. Burnout takes place when one's value structure leads to expectations which cannot be met by work. This type of analysis should not be taken as a way to diminish or dismiss the factors of dissatisfaction as unim-portant. Salary, relationship to one's peers, company policy, super-vision, and the comfort and safety of the working environment are quite essential to successful living. When the helping professional suffers from lack of work satisfaction and also from work dissatis-faction it is more than burnout—it is the disintegration of our hu-manity. However, professionals have numerous mixes of the "dis-satisfiers" and "satisfiers" and what mixes precede burnout is still an important issue. Teachers, social workers, nurses, ministers, priests, and rabbis all suffer from work dissatisfaction. The dissatis-fiers may be tolerated because we have prior knowledge of their existence and make our individual adjustments. However, when we do not have reasonable levels of work satisfaction combined with work dissatisfaction, then the burnout symptoms begin to appear.

A note on Herzberg: he does not discuss the possibility that cer-tain professional work ends in burnout. The long-term care givers of the dying and of the mentally disturbed and emotionally disad-vantaged may be prime candidates for this type of analysis. Herz-berg suggests that there is still some salvation if we look outside work for growth. Let's go a step further. B. F. Skinner, in his utopian novel *Walden Two*, has an ingenious way of allocating dis-tasteful work: simply reduce the number of hours one must work so that the people with distasteful jobs can grow in the hobbies they entertain after leaving work. In a less utopian situation this would also mean more sabbaticals and longer periods for rest and recuper-ation. At times, work with the dying and retarded can be quite up-lifting, but the combination of no possibility for promotion and no recognition, for instance, may bring on burnout. Skinner's trade-off is important only for those situations where the possibility of improving the satisfiers is remote or even impossible.

Herzberg's analysis of working and living also addressed two additional issues. The first concerned productivity and satisfying work. He seemed confident that productivity would increase if we expanded work to include intellectual and emotional growth. One notable exception is the Volvo automobile assembly plants in Sweden (*Newsweek* August 21, 1972). Volvo employed the typical American auto assembly line which created a high level of worker alienation. Workers responded with wildcat strikes, job changing, and absenteeism. Workers and managers then restructured the manufacturing process. Instead of the assembly line, small groups were organized which emphasized cooperative planning and the development of high level skills. However, Volvo soon realized that they could be more productive if they returned to the conventional assembly line methods. Nevertheless Volvo decided against reverting to the assembly line because workers and management insisted that productivity should not outweigh employees' satisfaction. In other words, tension exists between the need for higher productivity and job satisfaction. Contrary to Herzberg's analysis, jobs which have higher levels of satisfaction need not be justified on the grounds that productivity increases.

The second issue Herzberg's analysis failed to address was the relationship between ends and means. He viewed growth in the work place largely in economic and psychological terms, to the exclusion of political terms. We could, for instance, be engaged in personally meaningful work but produce goods and even services that are harmful. We must, therefore, appraise our work along two major dimensions: importance to the worker and benefit to society. Herzberg rightly drew attention to the dreadful working conditions of our lives but failed to emphasize that what we produce is also worthy of moral consideration. We must go beyond Herzberg's account of satisfying work and emphasize that our relationship to the consumer and client must be morally defensible. Nevertheless, we should keep in mind Herzberg's basic points: one, the elimination of scarcity should be a means toward growth, not an avenue to consumption, and, two, not all work experiences are of equal importance in determining worker alienation.

REFERENCES

Edelwich, J. 1980. *Burnout: Stages of Disillusionment in the Helping Professions*. New York: Human Sciences Press, p. 14.

Herzberg, Frederick. 1966. *Work and the Nature of Man*. New York: Thomas Y. Crowell, pp. 77-91.

McConnell, E.A. 1982. *Burnout in the Nursing Profession*. St. Louis: C.V. Mosby Co., p. 70.

Newsweek, August 21, 1972. "Manufacturing: The Assembly Team," p. 69.

Quinn, R. and Stains, G. 1979. *The 1977 Quality of Employment Survey*. Ann Arbor: The University of Michigan Press.

Burnout:
What Price Care Giving?

Maureen McCarthy

Human service workers, by definition, have jobs that entail responsibility to people, and the stressors multiply as the needs of clients are assessed (Ivancevich and Matteson 1980). To the question "Why did you select the mental health profession as a career field?" the response is inevitably "the challenge to work with people rather than to shuffle paper." However, coping with complex problems and diverse personality types, as well as filling out reams of forms, make stress the norm in this career.

Mental health workers, by training, are sensitized to the importance of listening to others, yet their "want-to-help" attitude may cause blind spots regarding personal burnout. In a random sample of staff employed at a mental health outpatient clinic, the findings show the attitude that "burnout happens to the other guy, not to me."

According to French and Caplan (1980), jobs on organizational boundaries involve high stress, while job rotation increases role ambiguity. A management decision that required mental health outpatient staff to serve on-call emergency/crisis intervention rotation emerged as the greatest stressor. The on-call staff person is on duty 24-hours-a-day for seven consecutive days. During the on-call week, staff have to juggle the schedules of their regular clients and produce quick assessments for court hearings, even when extreme fatigue is evident. Constructive suggestions for dealing with the problems that ensue may go unheeded under the guise that the system is working well, or the timing is not in line with organizational

Maureen McCarthy, PhD, Clinical Services Manager, Chesapeake Mental Health Services, North Chesapeake, VA.

objectives, or it is not cost effective. These excuses further escalate stress by stifling employee feedback (Flach 1977).

Clinicians responding to crisis situations are confronted by overreacting family members, who demand the situation be corrected, the family member be cured, but it be done the way they say. Crisis intervention, in 90 percent of cases, necessitates on-the-spot education regarding institutional commitment criteria. Even when the commitment process has been outlined for the family, rigid belief systems reinforce denial, e.g., "You represent a public agency and you can pick up and take away this family member." The ambivalence of families toward filing a commitment petition and attending the actual hearing is linked to their reluctance to look like "the bad guy."

The ideology or philosophy of an agency underscores its mission and goals. Difficulties arise when different agencies serving the same client perceive the problem and solution differently. In incest cases, mental health workers suggest a jail term may send a tough message to the perpetrator and provide affirmative support for the victim. Advocating against incarceration in the state prison system "to help maintain the family" is a posture that creates strain between agencies and is experienced as a significant stressor by mental health professionals.

Deinstitutionalization creates double bind situations in two ways: (a) there is unspoken pressure not to overuse the Community Service Board's bed utilization allowance at a state hospital; (b) there is a very real lack of adequate community resources, especially for the indigent and the chronically mentally ill population. Lack of resources implies greater effort, and, as Freudenberger and Richelson (1980) suggest, the harder we try, the more we impair our efficiency and invite burnout.

Boundary-spanning activities, which imply interaction with an working knowledge of other service delivery systems, is a major challenge to all mental health workers. Clarifying the mission, policies and procedures of mental health service to various courts, jails, hospitals, social service agencies, and educational systems is a continuously time-consuming task, due in part to staff turnover and intraorganizational changes at human services agencies. Gill's (1980) astute observations are relevant. First, "the greater number of people the professional person has to work with, the higher are his chances of burning out." Second, "it seems ironic that those who altruistically enter the helping professions are the ones likely to experience frustration and disillusionment."

Inappropriate referrals occur, in part, due to lack of adequate feedback on interagency transfer and occasionally due to a power issue. In the case of some court-mandated therapy, the client attends sessions but refuses any psychological involvement. Such situations raise ethical issues for clinicians because they know that therapy means changes in insight on the part of the client, not merely keeping attendance records. The stressor involves trying to convince a judge that his or her decision may not have been therapeutic.

The urgency of time and task is epitomized by production quotas. Strain is noticeable when high job demand and low decision latitude are operative. For example, clinicians are randomly assigned intake cases, which both prediction and experience have shown will result in poor follow through on the client's part. When too many such cases are in a clinician's case load, the clinician will worry about a negative performance appraisal and will begin to doubt his or her own professional skills. From a different perspective, Charlesworth and Nathan (1985) write "if there is a poor job skill mix or an ill-defined task, job satisfaction will suffer and productivity will wane."

In a period where budgets are tightening, issues focusing on reimbursement and insurance are central to therapy. Some clients engage in therapy with a private vendor until their insurance expires; then they are referred to a public agency. The intake clinician at the mental health center then has to deal with the client's anger at being referred when the insurance monies have run out. The client often believes that a public agency means inferior treatment. Conversely, public agencies are now seeing sicker people on an outpatient basis because of the lack of funds for inpatients.

Family members who are care givers sometimes send conflicting messages to the mental health worker. They seek help, yet when arrangements are made for them to commence respite care or family therapy, they refuse services. Without being able to step back and see family members locked into an enabling-denial stance, the mental health worker runs the risk of overinvolvement and burnout.

The expectations of the employee are not usually known by the organization and are rarely considered or solicited. Albrecht and Selye (1979) pointed out that a corporation or organization has three dimensions: the economic, the social, and the human. All are interrelated. Therefore, the stressors listed last by mental health workers actually are most significant in terms of burnout precisely because they transgress the three dimensions, as follows:

- low job status/prestige with correspondingly low salaries compared poorly with other career fields;
- ten to twelve days annual vacation time was seen as severely restrictive and hardly enough time to unwind;
- lack of perks, bonuses, and mental health days, and limited training/promotional opportunities cause some respondents to question "the reward" for better than average job performance.

Although all the respondents, including males and females, were committed to career goals, some were already planning career changes, such as pursuing consulting, university teaching, or real estate "within the next few years." The question one has to raise is this: If the initial career field was satisfying, why the switch?

Burnout often shows itself in ritualistic, compulsive, cynical, and negative behavior and in feelings of being exhausted or emotionally drained. Recognizing the symptoms, one can make the necessary changes to prevent burnout.

According to respondents, strong family and professional ties, regular feedback and occasional compliments for a job well done, rap sessions, participation in lunch hour aerobics classes, interagency forums, and peer pressure "to go home at 5:00 p.m." do much for personal survival.

Dealing with a problem after it becomes apparent is crisis management. Preventive management anticipates issues and actively elicits expression of employee concerns. It is an approach that challenges and develops people, and ensures an organizational climate that promotes wellness.

Values affect choices. Choices affect energies and goals. Mental health workers need to value themselves as persons by taking note of their successes, making special efforts to change routine and environment, taking heed of stress signals sent out by the body, and being aware of their feelings and priorities.

Burnout is a process. According to Cohen (1985), the primary public health enemy of the 1980s is chronic, degenerative disease. Stress and burnout are often dealt with through unhealthy behaviors — smoking, overeating, lack of exercise, and abuse of drugs and alcohol. Preventing burnout implies altering work habits and lifestyles so that healing and personal affirmation take place.

BIBLIOGRAPHY

Albrecht, K. & Selye, H. (1979) *Stress and the Manager*. Englewood Cliffs, NJ: Prentice-Hall, Inc.

Charlesworth, E. A. & Nathan, R. G. (1985) *Stress Management, A Comprehensive Guide to Wellness*. New York: Atheneum Co.

Cohen, W. S. (1985) "Health Promotion in the Workplace," *American Psychologist, 40*(2): 213-216.

Flach, F. (1977) *Choices: Coping Creatively With Personal Change*. New York: J. B. Lippincott Co.

French, J. & Caplan, R. D. (1980) "Organizational Stress and Individual Strain." In J. D. Adams (Ed.), *Understanding and Managing Stress*. San Diego, CA: University Associates, Inc.

Freudenberger, H. J. & Richelson, G. (1980) *Burnout*. New York: Bantam Books.

Gill, J. J. (1980) "Burnout." *Human Development, 1*(1): 21-27.

Ivancevich, J. M. & Matteson, M. T. (1980) *Stress and Work: A Managerial Perspective*. Glenview, IL: Scott, Foresman & Co.

Burnout:
Absence of Vision

Florence E. Selder
Anne Paustian

One nurse stated poignantly, "Burnout is when you are no longer effective and you no longer care." The symptoms of the phenomenon, labeled burnout, have been described as a complex, stress-related phenomenon that is characterized by a state of physical exhaustion and emotional depletion resulting from conditions at work (Freudenberger 1980; Maslach 1982). In this article, we argue that the experience of burnout results from a failure to live up to one's ideals. We believe that an ideal model is established in response to the uncertainty experienced by the provider of health care services. By establishing an ideal model(s), the health care provider precludes experiencing a passion for the commitments that initially characterized his/her practice. Passion, commitments, and vision are antidotes to the phenomenon described as burnout.

UNCERTAINTY

The complexity of serving clients and their families in health care systems today has great impact on nurses and other health care providers. There are new roles, new technology, and new models of delivering health care to the public. Societal, consumer, economic, and political forces strongly influence health care systems which in turn affect the individual health care provider. The individual nurse may not understand the specific factors that are in force.

Florence E. Selder, PhD, RN, is Associate Professor and Urban Research Center Scientist, University of Wisconsin, Milwaukee, WI. Anne Paustian is Graduate Student, University of Wisconsin, Milwaukee, WI.

The professional may be concerned about layoffs and limited support personnel or staff, and may not be aware of declining occupancy rates, changes in patterns of patients' admissions and discharges, and competitiveness among health care agencies in the marketing of services. These are issues that were not present or not addressed by health care providers until recently.

There is great uncertainty in health care systems. Hospitals as corporations are concerned about surviving. Some predict that the small community hospitals, as well as some large teaching institutions, will not survive. Traditional methods of health care delivery are in jeopardy. Newer health care models, predicted on business principles, are projected for the future. The majority of nurses are not educationally prepared in business or marketing strategies. The corporate approach to health care is antithetical to the philosophical tenets of health care. The individual nurse faces the current situation with a great deal of uncertainty.

Furthermore, there are issues that have not been addressed or even conceived as dilemmas prior to the rapidly changing advances of technology. Regrettably, the development of these advances frequently has occurred without consideration of their ethical and economical ramifications. For example, as a society, we have not figured out how to pay for high tech services for all our citizens. It is no longer economically feasible to legislate for federal support for heart and liver transplants, as we once did for kidney dialysis.

In addition, the greater physical and psychosocial health care needs of patients and their families, as well as many other problems over time, and the great number of new and changing health care provider roles, confound the situation. All of these factors serve to create or intensify the uncertainty that health care providers experience.

IDEAL CARE GIVER

One way health care providers respond to the uncertainty in their clinical setting is by attempting to reduce the ambiguity. They do this in a variety of ways. For instance, a social worker may rigidly follow the rules in an agency, refusing to allow for any flexibility in their application. Following the rules reduces the ambiguity or the uncertainty experienced in the situation. However, this behavior may not serve the patients. In nursing, an extreme example of following the rules is to enforce visiting hours even though someone may have traveled a great distance to see a gravely ill relative. Similarly, new clinicians are very uncertain in transition from students to practitioners and often will follow procedural manuals explicitly, not taking into account a patient's needs, physical limitations, personal and family situation, or numerous other variables that an expert clinician automatically considers.

A common means of reducing uncertainty is to create an image of the ideal care giver. The notion is that the ideal care giver would be able to handle the complexities of any clinical situation. The ideal is then regarded as a standard of perfection by which to measure oneself. However, the ideal can only exist in one's mind and one's performance can never equal the image of perfection.

The "ideal care giver" personality has been described as characterized by the beliefs that the individual must work hard all the time, must be everything to everyone, must always try to help if asked, must never be wrong, must always keep striving to improve, and must sacrifice personal needs to those of others. When the person doesn't feel comfortable or competent, and becomes uncertain as to the ability to perform, he or she may attempt to get more education, to become more technically proficient, to set job priorities better, or to become better organized as a means of reducing the discrepancy between the self and the ideal model. When these strategies don't work, and in fact compound the problem, the individual may create barriers with patients and their families and begin to separate from co-workers in an attempt to alleviate the discomfort of being uncertain in an uncertain environment.

We suggest that a person committed to an ideal is prone to burnout because it can control the individual, whereas, the person committed to a vision is guided by possibilities. A vision is the manner in which one sees or conceives of something. The individual health professional has a vision of what it means to be a nurse, a doctor, or a social worker. In contrast, an ideal, by its very definition, is always beyond a person's reach and, therefore, doesn't permit any possibility of achievement. The ideal is static and always beyond the ordinary and even the extraordinary reach of the person. We believe that burnout is the result of failure to fulfill one's commitment. For health professionals it is not that they lack commitment, but rather that they are unaware that the commitment has moved from one of a vision to one of a commitment to an ideal. They fail to make a distinction between their vision of what they want to be or want to accomplish and some ideal picture of what they should be.

Gradually, there may be a shift from a commitment to a vision to a notion of the ideal nurse, doctor, or social worker. This shift in perception is subtle, progressive, and damaging.

To illustrate, a nurse plans to teach a patient about diabetes mellitus and learns that he is being discharged immediately. The nurse committed to an ideal of how patient teaching should be conducted will experience failure in his/her nursing care. What *can* be accomplished will not look like the way it *should* be done, the ideal. The nurse committed to the vision that nurses make a difference in people's lives will decide to teach the essential items as well as provide the patient with resources, and to empower the person to manage his/her diabetes. Both nurses provide teaching and yet one nurse reports feeling bad about what she or he did or did not do and the other nurse reports a feeling of accomplishment. The distinction lies in the commitment of the nurses. One nurse is committed to the vision of what nursing is and what actions are necessary, in whatever the circumstances demand.

PASSION

A nurse who recently quit her job said, "Burnout is not the experience of having too much to do but rather it is not having the energy to do things you know you can do and not enjoying the things you used to love to do." Passion is a deep, overwhelming, powerful emotion. Passion is boundless enthusiasm. If passion is the experience of being alive at the moment, and that sense of life is characterized by commitment and vitality, then burnout may be viewed as the absence of passion.

Invariably, a turning point or benchmark in one's transition from a beginning practitioner to a mature, seasoned practitioner is a specific patient situation. Most professional persons can recall those patient situations in the clinical setting that caused a turning point in their practice. These turning points may facilitate or hinder professional development. The following stories illustrate the point:

The patient, Sarah, was a 28-year-old female diabetic, who had been admitted to a medical unit of a large private hospital for control of the diabetes, neuropathy, and electrolyte imbalance secondary to the disease. The primary nurse working with Sarah was a 22-year-old female with less than one year's experience in hospital nursing. In addition to the patient's physical problems, the psychosocial areas identified were loss of control, rejection related to decreased self-worth, and trouble coping with death. The care plan arose out of a multidisciplinary care conference, at which there was an opportunity for team members to share insights and feelings. The nurses, chaplain, social worker, and attending physician were involved.

The care plan was shared with the patient, who said she was grateful. Prior to this point she had been angry and noncompliant. Sarah was surprised to be allowed to contribute to her own care plan. Throughout hospitalization, she was able to verbalize anger with the staff about her deteriorating physical status, her depression, and the need to put up a brave front. She began to develop feelings of being close to her parents as they shared their feelings of regret and love for her.

The parents were encouraged to participate in the plan of care and they allowed themselves to be supported throughout their daughter's hospitalization. The mother was often tearful and shared her feelings about her daughter's repeated hospitalizations and the fear of her daughter's death. The doctor met with both parents and informed them of Sarah's impending death. The discharge plans were made to enable the patient to die at home as she had requested; however, she died in the hospital one week after a hypoglycemic seizure and coma.

A second situation concerns a patient called Randy. Randy was admitted to the unit and he also died. Randy was 22 years old and two years younger than the nurse. Randy's medical history was known to the nurse. When he was a senior in high school, he found a "lump in his neck" which the biopsy confirmed as Hodgkins disease, stage IIA. This carefree teenager did not feel "sick," so he stopped his treatment and would not take his medicine. When his

condition deteriorated, he went to Mexico with his parents for Lae-
trile treatments. He returned home with "a few weeks to live" and
both lungs filled with cancer. He experienced fainting spells, bleed-
ing, shortness of breath, and constant pain. His parents were terri-
fied by his symptoms, angry about the unfairness of life, and grieving about the suffering and impending death of their son.

Randy was brought to the hospital after hemorrhaging at home,
was admitted and declared a "No Code." The nurse was relieved
that Randy was not assigned to her team of patients, but was able to
spend time with him and his family. Toward the end of her shift he
coughed, hemorrhaged, and died. The hysterical mother came out
to the nurses' station and the entire nursing staff ran to his room.
But there was nothing to be done, so they mechanically straightened
up the room and prepared the body—crying, shocked, and disbe-
lieving. When the rest of the family arrived, there was a very painful, tearful viewing of the body. The nurses spent time with the
family, sharing the grieving process. Meanwhile, 15 minutes after
Randy died, there was another death on the floor.

Several issues surfaced for both nurses during this experience.
The following issues were identified: (a) dealing with the death of
someone close in age; (b) the right of the patient to participate in his
own health care; (c) the involvement of patient and family; (d) the
value of nursing and a multidisciplinary approach; (e) the vulnerability of all the health care team because of their involvement; and
(f) the need for support among the staff. Each of these items was
discussed and shared. The nurses were able to review the experiences with us.

As a "good nurse," Randy's nurse was thankful to have been
present so that the family did not have to deal with total strangers.
But, she reported it left her feeling numb, needing to escape, grieving and in pain, angry, exhausted, and drained. Afterwards this
nurse reported that she continued to feel physically and emotionally
"burned out" and felt very detached from her nursing. She reported
that there was much more that could be done for parents and since
she couldn't do it she would cut back her hours to part-time. She
was unable to become involved with cancer patients for several
months following this event and only after support and counseling
did she begin to work with these patients. Sarah's nurse reported

that she felt she was part of a team and believed her nursing care made a difference.

What is the distinction between the two nurses in these situations? As consultants, we were able to identify several factors that may have accounted for the different reactions of the nurses. One of these factors was that Sarah's nurse did not report having an "ideal" picture of what nurses did. She reported that what mattered in nursing was the ability to make a difference in a person's life or death. The second nurse believed that there was a successful way to die and reported that Randy's death was too sudden and his parents were unprepared for it. She also felt helpless as she had no contact with the other patient who died on the unit.

INTERVENTIONS

Since we believe that continuous and prolonged uncertainty is the basis for burnout, the most effective interventions are those that are directed at reducing uncertainty.

One means to reduce uncertainty is to offer information to health professionals about the phenomenon of burnout and its characteristics, prevention, and treatment. In service programs on burnout and stress management programs are useful. In these programs the presenter will name or label the phenomenon that the staff is experiencing. Simply defining and describing the phenomenon will greatly reduce uncertainty for the individual.* The person now has the ability to communicate to others what heretofore may have been a subjective, lonely experience.

Another group of strategies that we advocated in the treatment and prevention of burnout are self-management strategies. The essence of these strategies lies in the empowerment of the individual to be the source of personal welfare. These strategies enable the person to feel less uncertain and to have a sense of self-mastery. Since there are interpersonal, intrapersonal, and institutional factors that contribute to a person's experience of uncertainty, the individual is helped to see that, in spite of organizational factors and sys-

---

*Although the authors resist the use of burnout as a term, they recognize that naming an experience is a useful strategy.

tem problems, something can be done to minimize the impact of these variables. There are several relaxation techniques that participants may use to protect themselves from external demands and contribute to their health. Other individual strategies include good health, diet, exercise, a support system, and personal goal setting. The latter strategy is recommended, as it serves as a buffer against the stress that may be generated from too few or too many goals and from those goals that may be inappropriate in terms of one's long- and short-range objectives. An example of inappropriate goals is the nurse who is enrolled full-time in a graduate program and is working in a demanding, highly stressed position with much overtime required where there is little control over scheduling. This may be an inappropriate clinical placement, since graduate study requires a certain stability in scheduling to meet deadlines and study requirements. The nurse is at risk for developing burnout.

Practitioners could be assisted in examining belief system(s) that guide their personal action. Belief systems are similar to little boxes. If the physician has a belief system that professionals know all things and do all things right, he or she could get trapped into a box that doesn't permit the acknowledgment of mistakes, the requesting of assistance, and the sharing of personal concerns or fears. The physician is trapped by the belief system and is at risk for developing burnout.

In working with individuals who report burnout, we find certain personal commonalities that deserve to be addressed in terms of intervention. The "ideal" care giver should be able to do everything well and alone. There seems to be an inability for that person to engage other people's assistance in the direct and indirect management of care. For instance, nurses will mop a floor if a patient's safety is endangered, fetch drugs from the pharmacy if the patient needs them, call the doctor for the pharmacist, the radiologist, or the social worker, if these professionals request or expect it. The individual nurse in these instances can be taught to ask others to do some of these jobs or even to enroll or delegate others in achieving a desired goal. The "ideal" care giver can be taught that quality care does not rest totally with him or herself. Respecting oneself will greatly limit the tendency to be responsible for all things. When one values one's worth and one's own contribution, then one is less likely to assume that what others do is more important. One can allow others to help assume responsibilities.

One strategy that assists practitioners to maintain their commitment to a vision and not to an ideal is the provision of feedback. For instance, in critical care units that are characterized by high mortality rates, ever-demanding new technologies, and large number of personnel, there is a lot of uncertainty. In an effort to reduce the uncertainty, nurses may become technically proficient and they may distance themselves or create barriers against the parents and the young patient's family. Sande (1983) described an alumni day, which parents and children who were treated in a particular intensive care nursery were invited to attend. The event was planned to afford nurses and staff the opportunity to see what had happened to the children who had once been very sick. This intervention reduced uncertainty for the staff by confirming the differences they made in sick children's lives and by reminding them that not all these children died and that, even in children's chronic illnesses, there is progress. Simply put, nurses and staff received feedback. That feedback affirmed their vision that they could make a difference. The alumni day confirmed that these once desperately ill children could become healthy. It also confirmed that the children did not continue to suffer from the care that may have been regarded as traumatic and hurtful. In fact, the nurse and the child met in a totally different context, one that created satisfaction and sharing.

A more common strategy used to reduce burnout and/or to treat or prevent it is the use of small groups where members are able to compare and share. This process reduces uncertainty about the nature of burnout. The group process can make the individual experiences seem less ambiguous. By sharing, the participants have the opportunity to legitimize their needs, to shift their perception, to initiate changes in the organizational system, to name or describe their experiences, and to bring closure to clinical events that have been left unfinished. An example of bringing closure to an event is the case of a social worker who managed a child abuse case that was fatal for the child. In the group, he was able to ventilate, to review the management of the case, and to share his anger and his helplessness.

One last strategy that we use in working with health professionals is to recognize the distinction between passion and empathy. A client once said, "You have more passion than empathy. Empathy is to understand intimately my reality. You do that and you do more." The distinction for us is that passion is the underpinning of a commitment to make a difference in another's experience. It is the discovery of what would make a difference. It is not only the experience of the other. It is more than understanding.

In summary, if passion is the experience of feeling alive and engaged at the moment and that sense of life (e.g., boundless enthusiasm) is characterized by commitment to a vision, then burnout is the absence of passion, commitment, and vision. In caring for others, passion would be the joy of discovering. Confronting uncertainty within the context of passion yields a sense of spontaneity. Confronting uncertainty within the context of ideals can cause burnout.

BIBLIOGRAPHY

Freudenberger, H. J. (1980) *Burn Out: How to Beat the High Cost of Success.* New York: Anchor Press.

Maslach, C. (1982) *Burnout — The Cost of Caring.* Englewood Cliffs, NJ: Prentice Hall, Inc.

Sande, D. (1983) Preventing burnout in intensive care nurseries. *Pediatric Nursing, 9,* 364-368, 394.

IV. BURNOUT AND INSTITUTIONAL/AGENCY CENTERS

Burnout —
A Study of a Psychiatric Center

Irene G. Sullivan

Attention is increasingly being focused on the burnout phenomenon. Popular literature describing case studies and numerous clinical research studies attests to its prevalence in mental health and social service organizations, industrial plants and the business community. This paper examines the prevalence of burnout in Harlem Valley Psychiatric Center, which serves over 3,500 patients from the surrounding communities. The results of the study with which I was involved indicate that the staff was experiencing an early stage of burnout.

LITERATURE REVIEW

What Is Burnout?

Burnout has been plagued by confusion (Maslach 1981); there is no single definition of burnout that has been accepted as standard,

Irene G. Sullivan, EdD, CSW, is Instructor, Guidance and Counseling, Long Island University-Westchester Division. She is also in private practice, Irvington, NY.

with the result that a researcher must choose from many definitions to design a research study. Burnout has been defined as an exhaustion of physical and mental resources (Freudenberger 1980; Lamb 1979), spiritual collapse (Storlie 1979), loss of positive energy, flexibility and resourcefulness (Seiderman 1978), loss of touch with the meaning of work (Berkeley Planning Associates 1977), objectification of the skills of human interaction (Karger 1981), ecological dysfunction (Carroll and White 1981), tedium (Pines and Kafry 1978), and a syndrome of emotional, physical and attitudinal exhaustion and cynicism (Maslach and Jackson 1981). While there is no single, standard definition of burnout, there is general agreement that burnout occurs at an individual level; that it is an internal experience, usually psychological in nature, involving feelings, attitudes, motives, expectations; and that it is a negative experience that produces distress, discomfort, dysfunction, and/or negative consequences (Shinn 1981).

How Does Burnout Develop?

Researchers have identified burnout by symptoms and by stages, and many disagree over whether or not a consistent pattern emerges, and whether or not the process is gradual, infectious, erratic or dynamic. Burnout has been described as erratic and infectious (Seiderman 1978), having a subtle pattern that makes identification difficult (Mattingly 1977), a syndrome of responses identifiable by magnitude and frequency (Maslach 1978), a dynamic process (Cherniss 1980), a dynamic process with four stages of development (R. Daley 1979; Edelwich and Brodsky 1980; Costello and Zalkin 1963), and by identifiable symptoms that infect the whole staff (Munro 1980). There is general agreement that burnout occurs after the first year of one's career (as shown by a high rate of turnover), suggesting a lack of preparation for coping with the emotional stresses of the job (Barad 1979; Cherniss 1980; Freudenberger 1974; Lamb 1979; Maslach 1976; Maslach and Pines 1977). Those staying on the job experience an increasing degree of burnout the longer they stay in the mental health field (Pines and Maslach 1978). However, the oldest workers have a lower rate of both burnout and turnout

(Daly 1979), perhaps due to an ability to accommodate their expectations of themselves, their clients, and the system (Gardell 1976).

What Causes Burnout?

Burnout has been attributed to the individual, to the workplace, and to their interaction. Some researchers have concentrated on the failure of the individual system's unique struggle to achieve (Mattingly 1977); the individual who makes excessive demands on energy, strength or resources by trying too hard and aiming too high (Freudenberger 1975, 1980; Lamb 1979); exposure to stressors and frustrations which exceed the person's tolerance and coping resources (Carroll 1979); and the different motivations of individuals who work with patients, each motivation leading to its own particular form of stress (Vachon 1978). Other researchers have concentrated on the idiosyncratic nature of stress at work (Weinberg, Edwards, and Steinau 1979), and the lack of satisfiers in the environment (Pines and Kafry 1978). Several researchers have concentrated on the job that cuts the worker off from the authentic expression of his skills (Karger 1981), the frustrations in the work environment that lead to the progressive loss of idealism and energy which results in total disillusionment (Edelwich and Brodsky 1980), and the emotional, physical, and attitudinal exhaustion and cynicism which result from work related stresses involving intense, continuous interpersonal contact with other people (Maslach and Jackson 1981). Although the literature deals with the individual characteristics and behavior that cause burnout, and the interaction between the individual and the workplace, much of the literature concentrates on the organizational dimensions and interpersonal dimensions of the job that may make a person susceptible to burnout.

Job Dimensions

Skill variety is one dimension that taps the cognitive capacity of the individual and enhances challenge and interest in the work (Pines and Kafry 1978; Frankenhauser 1977). Variety is one of the core dimensions theoreticians specify as related to employee satisfaction, performance, and attendance (Dehlinger 1978; Frankenhauser and Gardell 1976; Gardell 1976, 1977; Hackman and Oldham 1974). Many professional and nonprofessional mental health workers experience identical feelings of alienation, frustration, apathy, powerlessness, meaninglessness, fatigue, attenuated self-worth, and social isolation due to a lack of challenge, underutilization of abilities and skills, and a paucity of intellectual stimulation in their work (Berkeley Planning Associates 1977; Cherniss 1980; Kermit and Kushin 1969; Pines and Maslach 1978).

Task significance, or the opportunity to view their jobs as having a substantial impact on the lives of other people, is related to job satisfaction, a sense of competence, and successful achievement (Maslach and Jackson 1981; Pines and Kafry 1978) by health professionals whose primary reason for entering their professions was to help people (Maslach 1978). Failure to see results and the belief that the work has no significance produces feelings of hopelessness, incompetence, lack of success, depression, dissatisfaction with the job, disillusionment, grief, anxiety, hostility, and physical and emotional exhaustion (Kermit and Kushin 1969; Maslach 1976; Maslach and Jackson 1981; Pines and Kafry 1978; Pines and Maslach 1978; Storlie 1979).

Autonomy and staff participation in decision making are related to job satisfaction, decreased role ambiguity, greater use of skills, goal clarity and attainability, better communication among staff, and a more positive sense of self (Cherniss 1980; Cherniss and Egnatios 1978; Pines and Maslach 1978; Seiderman 1978). While they may use highly formalized rules in avoiding overload and reducing uncertainty over role behavior in new workers, experienced workers locked into inflexible rules report feelings of powerlessness, alienation and isolation, frustration, mental strain, and burnout (Aiken and Hage 1966; Berkley Planning Associates 1977; M. R. Daley 1979; Frankenhauser 1977; Gardell 1976, 1977; Munro 1980; Pearlin 1967). Hierarchical power structures reduce staff autonomy and control and contribute to learned helplessness and burnout (Cherniss 1980).

Feedback that gives direct and clear information about the work itself is essential if workers are to gain knowledge of their performance levels and if they are to achieve a sense of significance and success. Lack of information about mental health workers' success and performance is significantly related to burnout (Maslach and

Jackson 1981; Pines and Kafry 1978). Large caseloads that prevent case resolution limit feedback and produce negative feelings that the counselors' work and agency are ineffectual (R. Daley 1979; M. R. Daley 1979; Freudenberger 1977; Mattingly 1977). Negative feedback from clients, whether justified or not, produces feelings of anger, fear, frustration, and incompetence (Kadushin 1974; Maslach 1978).

Role overload, both qualitative and quantitative, produces psychological and physical strain (French and Caplan 1973; Maslach and Pines 1977). Quantitative refers to having "too much to do," while qualitative means work that is "too difficult," but both are subjective and are influenced by the individual's personality and predispositions (Cooper and Marshall 1976). Although most studies do not differentiate between qualitative and quantitative overload, Caplan, Cobb, French, Harrison, and Pinneau (1980) report a significant relationship between qualitative overload and heart disease and lowered self-esteem. Other studies report a significant relationship between qualitative overload and stress; frustration; physical, mental and emotional exhaustion, and burnout (R. Daley 1979; M. R. Daley 1979; Kahn 1978; Storlie 1979; Vachon 1978, 1979). There is general agreement that overload increases moodiness and pressure on the job; it decreases competence, tolerance, satisfaction, creativity, and it produces negative attitudes and emotional detachment from clients, work and the workplace, and results in physical, mental, and emotional exhaustion.

Organizational Dimensions

Role clarity, leadership, and efficiency are the three major characteristics of organizations that have been identified as influential factors which cause workers to experience emotional exhaustion, depersonalization and lack of personal satisfaction (Cammann, Fichman, Jenkins, and Kelsh 1983; Cherniss and Egnatios 1978; French and Caplan 1973; Frankenhauser and Gardell 1976; Ilgen and Hollenback 1977; Cooper and Marshall 1976; Maloff 1975; Margolis 1974; Kahn et al. 1964).

Interpersonal Dimensions and Social Support

Co-workers and supervisors who have not provided support to workers have been found to be a source of stress and a contributing factor to burnout (Argyris 1964; Berkeley Planning Associates 1977; Cooper 1973; French and Caplan 1973; Kahn et al. 1964; Maslach and Jackson 1981). Programs in which supervisory support and leadership tended to result in lower levels of burnout among the workers during the first year on the job, while workers who worked under supervisors who were unavailable, dictatorial; and arbitrary experienced higher levels of burnout (Berkeley Planning Associates 1977). Although the evidence of the impact of social support on burnout from co-workers and supervisors does not appear to be consistent, most staff want supervisors to help them come to terms with their feelings and perceptions (Cherniss and Egnatios 1978b).

THE STUDY OF BURNOUT

A review of the literature on burnout has suggested that no single trait or single category of characteristics defines the cause of burnout, but that burnout seems to be the result of the interaction of several sets of variables. A decision was made to use the three sets of variables identified as evidence of burnout by the Maslach Burnout Inventory to study the prevalence of burnout at the psychiatric institution. Those characteristics of burnout described by Maslach (1981) include:

1. *Emotional exhaustion*. As emotional resources dwindle, workers grow less able to deal with their colleagues and their clients.
2. *Depersonalization*. Workers develop attitudes of dislike and cynicism toward their clients.
3. *Personal devaluation*. Workers rate themselves more and more negatively in terms of job performance.

A decision was also made to identify several sets of causes of burnout in the work environment to investigate whether or not any correlation existed between those sets and the characteristics of burnout described by Maslach. The variables included the job dimensions, organizational dimensions, and interpersonal support described in the literature review above.

To examine the impact of the work environment on burnout, a questionnaire was administered to 406 direct-care clinical staff representing nine staff positions. Four hypotheses were tested.

1. Negative job characteristics will correlate with burnout.
2. A lack of interpersonal supports will relate to burnout.
3. Negative organizational traits will have an impact on burnout.
4. The discrepancy between expectations and the impact of the work situation will relate to burnout.

THE RESULTS OF THE STUDY

The results of the study support the hypotheses of the relationship between burnout as characterized by the Maslach Burnout Inventory and the three sets of variables — job dimensions, organizational dimensions and interpersonal support.

The major correlates of emotional exhaustion in the area of job dimensions were the lack of influence in the work environment and the extent to which staff felt work overload. The other areas of the job dimensions — skill variety, task significance, feedback, and opportunities for personal development — were significantly related to feelings of personal accomplishment and feelings of depersonalization. The data supported the first hypothesis.

The major correlate of emotional exhaustion and depersonalization in the area of interpersonal support was the social support from one's supervisor. The need for support from one's co-workers was of less magnitude. The data supported the second hypothesis with regard to emotional exhaustion and depersonalization, but not with regard to personal accomplishment.

The major correlates of emotional exhaustion and depersonalization in the area of organizational dimensions was the lack of efficiency of the organization. The other areas of the organizational dimension — the worker's knowledge of what is expected from him/her and the leadership exhibited by supervisory personnel — were significantly related to emotional exhaustion and depersonalization.

The data supported the third hypothesis with regard to emotional exhaustion and depersonalization, but not with regard to personal accomplishment.

A significant relationship was found between emotional exhaustion and the extent to which the job met the staff's expectations. Significant correlates of emotional exhaustion and depersonalization were found in the discrepancy between the expectations and actual experiences of staff members with support from supervisors, the degree of leadership from supervisors, and the efficiency of the organization. The data supported the fourth hypothesis with regard to emotional exhaustion and depersonalization, but not with personal accomplishment.

CONCLUSION AND RECOMMENDATIONS

The results of the study supported the concept that there is a direct relationship between burnout and the organizational environment in which the worker spends the greater part of his day. The data revealed specific features of that environment that contributed to burnout of staff, i.e., work overload, lack of influence on the job, organizational inefficiency, and lack of supervisory support. The supervisor's support of the worker was found to be a mediating factor in minimizing the negative effects of the work environment and was recommended as a strategy to prevent burnout.

In order to minimize or prevent burnout of staff, several strategies were recommended. One strategy was the training of supervisors in management skills and worker relations. Another strategy involved the periodical reassessment of their work and their effectiveness on the job by all employees with the help of both supervisors and peers. Other strategies included training new workers to identify the characteristics of burnout and pointing out to new workers the realities of their job environment. That this study was carried out by the staff of the psychiatric institution may have influenced the absence of any recommendations submitted to administration that would review the problems of work overload, organizational inefficiency, and the sense the staff had that they lacked influence on their work environment.

REFERENCES

Aiken, M., and Hage, J. 1966. "Organizational alienation: A comparative analysis." *American Sociological Review, 31,* 497-507.

Argyris, C. 1964. *Integrating the Individual and the Organization.* New York: Wiley.

Barad, C.B. 1979. Study of burnout syndrome among Social Security Administration field public contact employees. Unpublished report. Washington, D.C.: Social Security Administration.

Berkeley Planning Associates. 1974-77. "Project Management and Worker Burnout," Final Report. (Volume IX) of the Evaluating Child Abuse and Neglect Demonstration Projects, U.S. Department of Commerce, National Technical Information Service.

Cammann, C., Fichman, M., Jenkins, D., and Kelsh, J. 1983. Chapter 9. Michigan Organizational Assessment Questionnaire. In S.E. Seashore, E.E. Lawler III, P.H. Mirvis, and C. Cammann (Eds.). *Assessing organizational change: A guide to methods, measures and practices.* New York: Wiley Interscience.

Caplan, R.D., Cobb, S., French, Jr., J.R., Harrison, R.V., and Pinneau, Jr., S.R. 1980. *Job demands and worker health: Main effects and occupational differences.* Ann Arbor: Institute for Social Research, University of Michigan.

Carroll, J. 1979. "Staff burnout as a formal ecological dysfunction." Unpublished paper presented at the *12th Annual Eagleville, Pa. Conference.*

Carroll, F., and White, W. 1981. "Understanding burnout: Integrating individual and environmental factors within an ecological framework." *Proceedings of the First National Conference on Burnout.* Philadelphia, Pa.

Cherniss, C. 1980. *Staff burnout: Job stress in the human services.* Beverly Hills, Calif.: Sage Publications.

Cherniss, C., and Egnatios, E. 1978a. "Is there job satisfaction in community mental health?" *Community Mental Health Journal, 14,* 309-318.

Cherniss, E., and Egnatios, E. 1978b. "Participation in decision-making by staff in community mental health programs." *American Journal of Community Psychology, 6,* 171-190.

Cooper, C. 1973. *Group Training for Individual and Organizational Development.* Basel, Switzerland: S. Karger.

Cooper, C., and Marshall, J. 1976. "Occupational sources of stress: A review of the literature relating to coronary heart disease and mental ill health." *Journal of Occupational Psychology, 49,* 11-19.

Costello, T., and Zalkind, S. 1963. *Psychology in Administration; A Research Orientation.* N.J.: Prentice Hall.

Daley, R. 1979. "Burnout: Smoldering problem in protective services." *Journal of Social Work, 24,* 375-379.

Daley, M.R. 1979. "Preventing worker burnout in child welfare." *Child Welfare, LVIII,* 443-450.

Edelwich, J., and Brodsky, A. 1980. *Burn-out: Stages of disillusionment in the helping professions.* New York: Human Sciences Press.

Frankenhauser, M. 1977. "Job demands, health and well being." *Journal of Psychosomatic Research, 21*, 313-321.

Frankenhauser, M., and Gardell, B. 1976. "Underload and overload in working life: Outline of a multidisciplinary approach." *Journal of Human Stress, 2*, 35-46.

French, J., and Caplan, R. 1973. "Organizational Stress and Individual Strain." In A. J. Marrow (Ed.), *The Failure of Success*. New York: AMACOM.

Freudenberger, H.J. 1974. "Staff burn-out syndrome." *Journal of Social Issues, 30*, 159-165.

Freudenberger, H. 1975. "The staff burn-out syndrome in alternative institutions." *Psychotherapy: Theory, Research and Practice, 12*, 73-82.

Freudenberger, H.J. 1977. "Burn-out: Occupational hazard of one child care worker." *Child Care Quarterly, 6*, 90-99.

Freudenberger, H.J. 1980. *The High Cost of High Achievement*. New York: Doubleday.

Gardell, B. 1976. "Technology, alienation and mental health. Summary of a social psychological research programme on technology and the worker." *Acta Sociologica, 19*, 83-93.

Gardell, B. 1977. "Psychological and social problems of industrial work in affluent societies." *International Journal of Psychology, 12*, 125-134.

Hackman, J.R., and Oldham, G.R. 1974. *Job Diagnostic Survey: An Instrument for the Diagnosis of Jobs and the Evaluation of Job Redesign Projects*. ERIC REPORTS, ED 099 580.

Ilgen, D., and Hollenback, J. 1977. "The role of job satisfaction in absence behavior." *Organizational Behavior and Human Performance, 19*, 148-161.

Kadushin, A. 1974. *Child Welfare Services*. New York: Macmillan Co.

Kahn, R. 1978. "Job burnout: Prevention and remedies." *Public Welfare*, 61-63.

Kahn, R., Wolfe, D., Quinn, R., Snoek, J., and Rosenthal, R. 1964. *Organizational Stress: Studies in Role Conflict and Ambiguity*. New York: Wiley.

Karger, A. 1981. "Burnout as alienation." *Social Service Reviews*, 12-19.

Kermit, I., and Kushin, F. 1969. "Why high turnover? Social staff losses in a county welfare agency." *Public Welfare*.

Lamb, H. 1979. "Staff burnout in work with long-term patients." *Hospital and Community Psychiatry, 30*, 396-398.

Maloff, B. 1975. "Peculiarities of human service bureaucracies." *Administration in Mental Health*, 36-45.

Margolis, B. 1974. "Job Stress: An unlisted occupational hazard." *Journal of Occupational Medicine, 16*.

Maslach, C. 1976. "Burned-out." *Human Behavior, 5*, 16-22.

Maslach C. 1978a. "Job burn-out: How people cope." *Public Welfare, 36*, 56-58.

Maslach, C. 1978b. "The client role in staff burn-out." *Journal of Social Issues, 34*, 111-124.

Maslach, C. 1981. "Understanding burnout: Problems, progress and promise." *Proceedings of the First National Conference on Burnout*. Philadelphia, Pa.

Maslach, C., and Jackson, S. 1981. "The measurement of experienced burnout." *Journal of Occupational Behavior, 2,* 99-113.

Maslach, C., and Pines, A. 1977. "The burn-out syndrome in the day care setting." *Child Care Quarterly, 6,* 100-113.

Mattingly, M. 1977. "Sources of stress and burn-out in professional child care work." *Child Care Quarterly, 6,* 127-137.

Munro, J. 1980. "Preventing front-line collapse in institutional settings." *Hospital and Community Psychology, 31,* 179-182.

Newman, J., and Beehr, T. 1979. "Personal and organizational strategies for handling job stress: A review of research and opinion." *Personnel Psychology, 32,* 1-43.

Pearlin, L. 1967. "Alienation from work: A study of nursing personnel." In M. Abrahamson (Ed.), *The Professional in the Organization.* Chicago: Rand McNally.

Pines, A., and Kafry, D. 1978. "Occupational tedium in the social services." *Social Work,* 499-507.

Pines, A., and Maslach, C. 1978. "Characteristics of staff burnout in mental health settings." *Hospital and Community Psychiatry, 29,* 233-237.

Pines, A., Aronson, E., and Kafry, D. 1980. *Burnout.* New York: The Free Press.

Seiderman, S. 1978. "Combatting staff burn-out." *Day Care and Early Education,* 6-9.

Shinn, M. 1981. "Caveat emptor: Potential problems in using information on burnout." *Proceedings of the First National Conference on Burnout.* Philadelphia, Pa.

Storlie, F. 1979. "Burnout: The elaboration of a concept." *American Journal of Nursing,* 2108-2111.

Vachon, M. 1978. "Motivation and stress experienced by staff working with the terminally ill." *Death Education,* 113-122.

Vachon, M. 1979. "Staff stress in care of the terminally ill." *Quality Review Bulletin,* 13-17.

Vachon, M., Lyall, W., and Freeman, S. 1978. "Measurement and management of stress in health professionals working with advanced cancer patients." *Death Education, 1,* 365-375.

Weinberg, E., Edwards, G., and Steinau, R. 1979. Burnout among employees of state residential facilities serving the developmentally disabled. Unpublished manuscript.

Is Burnout
an Institutional Syndrome?

William Weiner

Federal institutions are often accused of having a poor appraisal and reward system for their employees, which can lead to disillusionment, apathy, alienation and, consequently, burnout. This essay will point out some of the shortcomings of the system and some of the reasons for the shortcomings. However, the main emphasis will be on the individual and his or her particular response to a seemingly uncaring and unresponsive environment.

One of the reasons an institution has a noncaring attitude toward its employees is that it tries to uphold the values of the larger societal system. Status quo in this perspective could then be seen as a top priority, sometimes at the expense of the employees. Maintaining the status quo may not permit individuality and creativity since they may deviate from the current norm and may be seen as threatening to the system. Not having ideas realized and implemented can lead to despair in the person who is not recognized for who he or she is and who feels unable to make an impact on his or her organization. The reason federal institutions seem to lack rewards for their employees may also be due to the stoic view that excellence and competence are expected and need no reaffirmation. Tied in with this notion is the old-fashioned, out-dated view of Rank's "Trauma of Birth" (p. 319 in Wolman 1960) in which learning takes place through suffering. While this orientation may be very subtly used, the message is that the individual has to come to terms with the demands made by the federal system, i.e., the individual has to uphold its value system without demanding any reward or support

---

William Weiner, ACSW, is affiliated with the Department of Social Services, Bronx Veterans Administration Hospital, Bronx, NY.

95

for it. The suffering involved comes from relinquishing positive feedback, a human need without which the individual may question his or her own value.

Edelwich and Brodsky (1980) propose a useful model of the stages of disillusionment leading to burnout:

1. *Enthusiasm*. The individual has unrealistic expectations of his or her job and becomes overinvested in it to make up for personal disappointments and shortcomings.
2. *Stagnation*. The person becomes aware that the job is not quite what he or she imagined it to be and cannot make up for whatever is missing in his or her personal life.
3. *Frustrations*. The person feels the disappointments and limitations of the job, and begins to question his or her own competency and the reason for remaining in this particular field or profession.
4. *Apathy*. This is a defense against chronic frustrations.

The authors add "Intervention" in order to avoid burnout. Intervention, which causes the individual to make some changes, can take place anytime but is most successful in the first stage of "Enthusiasm."

I find this model helpful because burnout is seen as the result of disappointments and disillusionment with the environment and with the self. However, temporary setbacks and disappointments are not necessarily part of the burnout syndrome. Rather, they should be seen as part of a process enabling the curious person to make changes in his or her life and job as needed. He or she would not feel the helpless victim in any situation.

As the term burnout implies, there is a barren feeling due to a traumatic event with little or no hope for change. The individual who is not at that stage will have a much more realistic approach to his or her job, since his or her life and satisfaction do not depend on having all or most needs met by the institution. The level of enthusiasm is based on good feelings about the self, and self-esteem does not require the fulfillment of unrealistic expectations to fill a deadness or void in life. One of the criteria of a "well-adjusted person" would be the ability to solve problems successfully in most situations and to come to terms with limitations imposed by a specific job. This person would recognize the options open to him or her and make the appropriate choice in his or her own best interest.

I would define the last stage of apathy as a life-style rather than an attitude toward a current work situation. As mentioned earlier, Edelwich and Brodsky describe apathy as a defense against frustration. My own view and orientation is that apathy is the unsuccessful attempt at coping by the individual who feels overlooked and rejected by the situation. However, in order to see the reasons for apathy, one has to look back to unresolved childhood experiences. The person who felt unrewarded and unappreciated for who he or she was in childhood is much more vulnerable to uncaring responses in the environment. As a matter of fact, not being appreciated by the institution may validate his or her earlier experience. The apathy that manifests itself in such an individual as lack of emotion, lack of interest, indifference, lethargy, etc., which are all part of burnout, is the always present, though sometimes dormant, past of this individual's personality and life-style.

It has been said that dependent people tend to seek civil service jobs. Such people look for a strong father figure for care and protection. They rely on others for their security and well being, but their need for independence causes great anxiety in them. Giving up one's individuality, even in the dependent person, can lead to frustration and apathy.

A person with an unrealistic ego-ideal is also subject to burnout. This individual has expectations of himself or herself that are impossible to live up to. Unable to realize his or her goals, the person becomes frustrated and either blames the institution for not recognizing his true value or blames himself or herself for not being good enough to achieve his or her goals. The person has set very high standards in order to win approval and recognition from others. This individual will settle only for perfection and when this is not attainable, will have all the symptoms of the burnout syndrome. Unrealistic expectations of oneself and the need for perfection in order to please others are rooted in very early life events.

Social workers out of graduate school are usually very enthusiastic about being mental health professionals and look forward to helping people with their emotional problems and to intervening in their environmental situations when necessary. This might include financial assistance, housing, home care, etc. However, the enthusiasm soon subsides when faced with the reality of many situations. Social workers in institutional settings who see themselves as "therapists" soon find their caseloads to be very great while many other demands are made of them. While doing individual, couples, and group therapy is always encouraged, the demands and primary goal of the institution are rarely in tune with the social workers'.

Priorities in a hospital setting would include discharge planning, which, for the most part, consists of supplying concrete services such as home care, housing, and financial assistance. Discharge planning does require counseling regarding acceptance of illness by the patient and family, dependency on the hospital, marital and family conflicts, etc. However, discharge has to occur according to a time table and, more often than not, the problem presented cannot be worked through completely within the prescribed time frame. The social worker, due to other commitments, may also not be able to spend as much time as needed with a particular case. The required home care, housing, and financial assistance may not be available at the time of discharge either because of ineligibility or lack of time. The social worker who started out with a spurt of enthusiasm now finds, to a great extent, that he or she really cannot accomplish what he or she set out to do. The patient may at times complain to the worker or the supervisor that help is not forthcoming. "You are the social worker; how are you helping me?" is often heard when, in reality, no "real" help may be available except empathy and understanding. While the therapeutic stance here is that the patient is really talking about his frustrations caused by health problems, financial difficulties, etc., the gnawing doubt in the social worker remains that "there should be more that I could do than just to understand how he feels in these very difficult and trying circumstances." The social worker may feel helpless and unappreciated by his patient for the efforts exerted in trying to help the patient and may begin to question his or her own competence and reason for being in the field. Disillusioned, he or she turns to the institution for moral support. More often than not he is not heard or given credence. (If he persists he will be labeled as suffering from burnout and asked to shape up or ship out.) Unheard and unappreciated for who he or she is and what he or she is trying to accomplish, the worker's attitude may deteriorate further.

The social worker with great dependency needs, as mentioned

before, will experience further disillusionment when confronted by a dependent patient. Not only are his or her needs not met but, to compound his or her own frustrations, he or she is up against the unrealistic dependency needs of others.

Another issue leading to disappointments is accountability, which is of major concern to the institution. This involves heavy loads of paperwork and statistical data to prove the need for social work involvement. Social workers as well as other professionals have a hard time accepting what they view as time wasting tasks. They feel infantilized and they feel they have to spend a great deal of time doing things that are not worthy of their professionalism and educational background.

Another burnout issue for social workers in a hospital setting is the hierarchical system in which the medical model has top priority. "Real help," according to this view, can only come from a physician. Patients who are a product of this culture also believe that the more prestigious physician is the only one qualified and able to help them. Although social service has many important functions, such as appropriate discharge planning and counseling, which may well determine the future health and well-being of an individual, it plays a secondary role in the hospital and social workers are only called in after the doctor is finished with the patient. The person with low self-esteem may take this as a personal affront, may think he or she is considered a second-class citizen.

The question is whether it is possible to change the system or whether the individual can be taught how best to cope in a seemingly unresponsive environment. While it is true that we all need positive reinforcement, it is also true that this would be most crucial in the first years of life. The person who had "good mothering" to begin with may not get caught up in the defensive maneuvering required by the institution. The individual who is able to understand and empathize with institutional regulations will fare much better than the person who sees them as affronts to his or her integrity and responds negatively to their demands. The social worker is usually in a key position to help patients and their families with discharge planning and is responsible for the future successful adjustment in the environment. Thus, even though the social worker does not hold the prestigious medical degree which is most valued in the system, he or she can still derive satisfaction from a job well done, secure in his or her own individual contribution.

The literature on burnout is very clear as to how the job affects the individual. What is not spelled out clearly is the input of the individual. Is he or she, in fact, mostly a passive recipient with few choices or does he or she have a say in the matter? It would seem to me that how the individual responds to any given job situation tells us more about the individual than about the environment.

Thus, in ending, I would like to offer a model for understanding disillusionment leading to burnout. This process-focused model views disillusionment on a continuum. Running parallel to this continuum would be the person's inner experience of his total self, as related to work and to personal life. That is, if his or her private life were satisfying, it seems possible that, despite the impact of disillusionment at any one point, his or her integrity would be preserved. The total process of burnout at any stage of disillusionment would be shrugged off and handled as an outside force, leaving little imprint on the person's sense of total self. It is hoped that this awareness of both the person as an individual, and the institution as a system, would lead to an appreciation and acceptance of each. Harmony within the self and between the self and the system might then replace burnout as a more rewarding, unified experience.

REFERENCES

Edelwich, J. and Brodsky, A. 1980. *Burn-Out.* New York: Human Sciences Press.

Kohut, H. 1984. *How Does Analysis Cure?* (Ed.: Goldberg, A. and Stepansky, P.E.) Chicago: The University of Chicago Press.

Mahler, S.M., Pine, F. and Bergman, A. 1975. *The Psychological Birth of the Human Infant.* New York: Basic Books, Inc.

Wolman, B.B. 1960. *Contemporary Theories and Systems in Psychology.* New York: Harper & Row.

V. COMBATTING BURNOUT

Rekindling the Flame:
A Self Psychology View of Burnout

Marcella Bakur Weiner

Burnout is often reported by professionals and linked to underlying feelings of apathy or lack of enthusiasm, a lack of connection to others and to one's work and a general "dead-end," "no-exit" state. Insightful interpretations such as Freudenberger's suggest that this syndrome occurs particularly in high achievers. In searching for a personal frame of reference within which to lodge this phenomenon, I have used the works of the late Heinz Kohut, the founder of Self Psychology, as applied to three particular areas of work: psychotherapy, consultancies, and teaching.

PSYCHOTHERAPY

One of Kohut's basic tenets (Kohut 1982) involves the concept of empathy. He interpreted empathy as a data-gathering tool enabling a psychotherapist to place him/herself inside a patient's self-state in order to understand it. In so doing, the goal of the therapist was to

Marcella Bakur Weiner, EdD, is Adjunct Professor, Fordham University Graduate School of Social Work at Lincoln Center, New York, NY.

internalize the sensitive, growth-supporting person, termed the "self-object," the patient never really had as a child. This internalization would, it was hoped, eventually lead to better self-esteem and good mental health in the patient. Empathy per se, i.e., the mere presence of empathy, would have a beneficial, therapeutic effect both in the clinical setting and in human life in general.

When "burnout" occurs in the psychotherapy process, the clinician experiences a helpless deadness. The "no-exit" feeling takes over and the label of either "negative therapeutic reaction" or "counter-transference problems" is used as a sealer or soother.

Self psychology would suggest that the formidable "negative therapeutic reaction" posited by Freud may be an understandable defense used by the patient to protect him/herself against disillusionment. Should this disillusionment occur, the patient is convinced, from past experience, that irreversible fragmentation of the self will take place. The therapist who can immerse him/herself into the patient's subjective reality can realize this terror empathically and will not necessarily feel a terrible transferential rejection or hopelessness at the patient's understandable dread of trusting once again. Rather, he will be able, patiently and most delicately, to provide the empathic understanding of the patient's narcissistic rage. Instead of an interpretation of "you are angry at me," offered confrontationally, he/she will accept and understand that anger or rage as the deep terror it is of abandonment-once-more taking place in the patient's life.

Removing the perhaps pejorative label of "negative therapeutic reaction," self psychology, the approach I have found most useful, suggests that the process taking place is in actuality a lack of attunement, or an empathic failure, on the psychotherapist's part. This leads to a revival of an old injury to the cohesion of the self in the patient, proving once again to the child, and now to the adult, how insensitive his original self-objects were to his feelings. Once again, the adult needs and does not get a mirror of his/her ambitions and achievements and the omnipotent ideal a child needs in order for idealization of the parent to take place from his/her environment, in this case his/her therapist. When the therapist offers him-herself as the good self-object the patient never had, he or she supplies a second chance. In short, what the psychotherapist offers to the patient is a second chance to believe in and then to internalize this good, reliable self-object. This may become a major area of conflict in the treatment and one of the most disheartening counter-transference feelings for the therapist, i.e., that he/she has not had any effect at all!

I have found, since using a self psychology approach, that this framework helps deal with impasses — including the burnout experienced by the therapist — which have produced therapeutic failures where there might have been successes. This view calls upon the therapist to ponder continually the impact of his/her intervention and to explore this impact if it seems to have distanced the patient. The therapist is called upon to set aside interpretive approaches that make the patient feel misunderstood, often triggering dangerous regression. This involves the sometimes difficult admission on the therapist's part that his or her interpretation (or, sometimes, what is experienced as a moralistic attitude) is off the track in the sense that it makes the patient feel indicted rather than empathically understood. An approach such as self psychology may lift both the sense of blame the patient feels as a result of a negative interpretation and the sense of helplessness and frustration the therapist feels, often called "burnout."

CONSULTANCIES

Idealization is most often realized in the form of love. How poignantly this is expressed can be felt in a famous love poem of Elizabeth Barrett Browning (1850):

> If thou must love me, let it be for naught
> Except for love's sake only. Do not say,
> 'I love her for her smile — her look — her way
> Of speaking gently, — for a trick of thought
> That falls in well with mine. . . .
> For these things in themselves, Beloved, may
> Be changed, or change for thee, — and love,
> So wrought,
> May be unwrought so. . . .
> But love me for love's sake, that evermore
> Thou mayst love on, through love's eternity.

Love suggests both idealization and a sense of infinite time. When love falters, it is that idealization has been replaced by criticism. Translated into analytic terms, the child who desperately wants to know that "you will be there when I need you; I can count on your strength and your caring when I feel in despair and helpless" is providing himself with an ideal figure, a staunch figure, one who will not fall apart under the stresses of life. This is also a figure who will be attuned to the child's emerging manifestations of his central self, i.e., an idealized parent will be interested in the child's interests, and will help him/her to begin to act on these interests.

Professionals who choose to be consultants often encounter idealization. The consultant is called in and paid well to preserve the infantile paradise we all long for! As a first-class problem-solver, he/she is looked upon to make the world right again, to turn chaos into order, to pour stable concrete into bottomless potholes and, basically, to make life livable for the clients. His/her grandiosity and omnipotence are sought after, reinforced, and soothed repeatedly by compliments and money and are seen as characteristics to be emulated by others. The general feeling among staff is: "The consultant is here. Everything will now be solved." At least, some of this has been my experience in my work as consultant to agencies.

"Burnout" in this situation simply does not appear. Conversely, "burnin" appears in the form of a flame inside the self which responds to an admiring, idealizing audience. One can almost do no wrong, for to do wrong would imply that those who hired the consultant were at fault—money was uselessly if not foolishly spent and heads would roll. The field is ripe for the consultant to be idealized just as the parent who is sensitive to the child at each crucial stage of development is idealized. Whereas the patient may "de-idealize" the therapist, as examined in the section on psychotherapy, this does not usually happen to the consultant. Rather, the converse operates. Peers look to the consultant as the expert. The consultant's dictums are transcribed forever into the field of work, enshrined and encased as much as the footprints of Hollywood stars. Since every moment is a highly-paid one, "the truth" must be uttered quickly, solutions speedily spelled out and goals solidly implemented. Burnout? Never. Like good wine, the intoxication is subtle but powerful! Its effects last a long time.

Because of the admiring audience, mirroring, as a concept developed by Kohut in the theory of self psychology, also takes place. Simply put, this involves an appreciation for one's accomplishments and one's sense of self. This can be easily seen to occur in the consultant. Unlike the situation in psychotherapy where, if disharmony between therapist and patient take place, the reason may be that they have different goals, consultants have goals similar or the same as those of the staff working with them—simply, to solve the problem or get things going again. Harmony has to reign even though the setting is "top-heavy" or authoritarian in nature, with the expert as the predominant player! And so, perhaps "burnout" does not occur in the consultant who is idealized. As in love, this can take place for some time, under special conditions, if the idealization is agreed upon by all—the person being idealized and those doing the idealizing!

TEACHING

What about teaching? Since many professionals practice therapy, do consultant work and also teach, it may be interesting to explore the dimensions of teaching as related to both burnout and self psychology. It would seem as though the act of teaching, whether on a graduate or undergraduate level, has some of the characteristics of both therapy and consultancies, but in different ways.

Idealization is a potential. Students have chosen, or been advised, to take a course with you. Students read the course description and expectations are clear: "I will take this course with you and you will teach me the XYZs described." The potential for idealizing the teacher is inherent. You are excited and waiting to fulfill expectations. Yet, the potential for de-idealization is also great. Students, even in a single classroom setting, are not homogeneous. While an individual psychotherapy can make sensitive contact with the subjective world of the patient, it is far more difficult to do so with two or three dozen students. Your idealization-thermostat waivers and burnout lurks in the wings. Idealization needs constant attention and focusing, just as lovers adore each other and caress and focus upon one another with intensity. But, is this true in the teaching situation? While your students are yours and for one or one-and-a-half hours look only to you for *"the truth,"* there are others to be reckoned with, such as deans, departmental chairs, administrators, assistant administrators and, above all, executive secretaries.

While your students may idealize you, that undermining agent of love—criticism—may be on the agenda for you! Your grading curve, some say, may be "too normal," "too extreme," etc. You may be considered demanding, for example, when you ask for a window in *your* classroom/office when windows are scarce, and so on. You may be viewed as infantile or needy in wanting a salary raise, another schedule, other courses, a parking place for your car, chalk for your blackboard . . . the list is endless. Your idealization, shored up within each teaching session, with rapt young (and sometimes older) faces opening up to you like beautiful vases waiting to receive flowers, may be shattered by the authority figures and/or peers with whom you work in the teaching setting. Unlike the consultant who is often hired under noncompetitive conditions, your skills, talents, and knowledge as a teacher can be easily replaced. Aware of this, you look to your students for more and more idealization because, in a time of crisis, fighting against burnout, *you* may need to turn to *them*, almost in a parent-reversal scenario, to reinstate you in the eyes of "the system." They, like the good parent, will have to defend you, fight for you, plead with the authorities to let you continue to do your job. How much of idealization is needed to counteract the possible influence of burnout due to administrative demands? How much sensitive attunement from parent to child and child to parent is needed to allow for the vicissitudes of life and to find life still beautiful and exciting? We don't know.

AGGRESSION:
A HOPEFUL VIEW

Another basic tenet of self psychology is the view of aggression as espoused by Kohut. Rather than seeing aggression as an innate drive, self psychology focuses on aggression as a disintegration product of an unresponsive environment. Not an untameable instinct, it can be examined within this framework as a reaction to an uncaring environment, situation, person or persons. In interpreting the aggressive drive in this way, perhaps there are clearer ways of perceiving hope. People need not feel trapped by the drives and instincts over which they have no control and therefore feel no hope. Self psychology offers optimism instead of pessimism. Burnout is the state of "no hope," when one feels that there is no way out of a situation. One feels tired and blames one's self for everything. Burnout, understandably, has components of depression. Why else the hopelessness and despair? Yet, if one were to understand that this phenomenon occurs *only* under certain conditions, one could have more control. One could hope for change. Seen in this context, self psychology, offering the understanding of the necessity for healthy idealization, empathy as a way of working with our patients, peers, family, and others, and seeing healthy grandiosity and healthy narcissism as positive aspects, may lead to a better grasp of dreaded burnout.

BIBLIOGRAPHY

Browning, E. (1850) Sonnets from the Portuguese. In: Untermeyer, L. *A Treasury of Great Poems*. New York: Simon and Schuster, p. 800.

Freud, S. (1923) Negative therapeutic reactions. *Standard Edition*. London: Hogarth Press, *19*, 49-50, 1961.

Freudenberger, H.J. (1980) *Burnout*. New York: Doubleday & Co.

Kohut, H. (1977) *The Restoration of the Self*. New York: International Universities Press.

Kohut, H. (1982) Introspection, empathy and the semicircle of mental health. *International Journal of Psychoanalysis, 63*, 395-407.

Weiner, M.B. and White, M.T. (1986) Uncooperative patients or empathic failures? A self psychology perspective. *Clinical Gerontologist*, Vol. 6, No. 2, p. 61-71.

White, M.T. and Weiner, M.B. (1986) *The Theory and Practice of Self Psychology*. New York: Brunner/Mazel, Inc.

A Day with Our Feelings

T. Earl Yarborough

Have you ever taken a moment of your time to stop and think about yourself? Those of us in the human service field always think about that special person and that special family we are serving, and this is the way it should be. Too few of us take enough time to pause to think about how we are living and whether our lives are really good. If we are to continue to commit our lives to serving other people, we have no choice but to pause, catch our breath, and think about our own personal lives. After all, each of us is an important person.

I have just completed 40 years in the field of funeral service. I hope to continue to serve families for many more years because I feel that I have never worked a day in my life. I love the field of service I am in because I feel I walk with a family through the most painful situation they will ever experience. Most people who are sincerely committed to a human service field feel the same way. Each of us loves people so much, and, when they are hurting, we must be there to lend a helping hand.

How do you feel when your day is over and you come home? What are your feelings about that day? Do you feel a lot of stress? Do you feel good about your day? Or are you disturbed and completely burned out? Do you ever say, "What a hell of a day I have had!" Maybe this is a true statement. This is especially true in my field of service when we have just served the family of a darling little child who has died. A perfect example is when a little child runs out in the street and is hit by a car. This just burns me out very quickly. But that loving family must go through the grief, and we

T. Earl Yarborough is Vice-President, Funeral Service, Harry & Bryant Co., Charlotte, NC.

must be with them. They need all of us beside them, and this is my life's commitment and the commitment to my God.

How do I handle this when the day is over and I come home? How do I work off the stress? Let me assure you that it isn't an easy thing to do.

Usually, when I get home, I change my clothes immediately. I put on a bright sport shirt and head for my back yard. My wife and I made an agreement years ago that I would take care of the yard and she would take care of the inside of the house. During the beautiful spring, summer, and fall seasons, I get my garden hose and water all the flowers, grass, and shrubs. If my two grandchildren drop by to see me, we always turn the hose on each other. This is fun, playing with Matt and Katie. I really enjoy being in our yard, and it is such a great release. Let me assure you that I am the world's best watering man. The flowers may be drowned about three times a summer because of my watering, but it is fun for me and it works off the stress at the end of the day.

Now when winter comes, it is even more peaceful and beautiful to me. When I get home, I change clothes, and that bright sport shirt is always there. Nothing in this world is as beautiful and peaceful to me as my fireplace. On a cold winter night, it makes me relax to cuddle up in my special chair with a good book.

The second most relaxing thing for me is my stereo system. I love beautiful music. Of course, I grew up in the big band era, and I still love that special music. Nothing is as relaxing to me as the music of Glenn Miller, Harry James, and Benny Goodman. Also, if you haven't heard Linda Ronstadt's "What's New" record, you are missing a great talent. By bedtime I am a relaxed, peaceful, and happy person. I never have any trouble sleeping. My evening prayer is simply this, "God, I have lived this day to the best of my ability, so let me rest in peace this night. Tomorrow, I will continue to live and serve people as you have taught me."

What is your attitude toward your feelings? Is your attitude toward life a positive attitude or are you a negative person? I hope you are a positive and an optimistic person. Let me assure you that this will make life so different for you.

Let me share with you some creative changes which some people have found could bring happiness back to their lives. Some of these ideas might be helpful to you in your search for relieving distress, to turn the tables on stress and to make it work for you, rather than against you.

We can really develop a healthy attitude if we think positively. I hope that each of us will learn to accept what we cannot change and love ourselves. We should never be afraid of failure, and we should practice living in the present.

In order for our bodies to have some strength, we must learn to relax, get a lot of rest, exercise, and dress in a way that makes us feel good.

We can improve our personal relationships by having a few good friends and several congenial acquaintances.

As we face painful situations, we should always work toward deepening the meaning of our lives. We should keep things in proper perspective and learn to let painful things go. Nothing is more meaningful to me than private time for meditation, to think about how I feel. Just letting go is so great, and it always encourages gentleness. Just don't try to be a perfect person, because no one can be.

To live a healthy life-style, just be yourself and take life as it is and your problems one at a time. As you think about your stress and problems, where do you go to release and dump the garbage?

One day a man walked into our funeral home, a man I had known for many years, and asked to see me. I took him into an office and closed the door. He immediately sat down in a chair and started crying. Without saying a word to me, he cried for about fifteen minutes as hard as any person could cry. After a while, he stopped crying, went into the bathroom and washed his face, and came back into the office and sat down. Then he said, "Earl, my wife is dying with cancer and I pass this funeral home every day on my way to the hospital. I have known you for many years, and I stopped in to see you this morning because this is the only place in Charlotte that I can cry and people will understand my feelings." Then he thanked me for the time I had spent with him and walked out of the door to visit his wife in the hospital. This man knew where he could go to release some real stress, and he knew how to handle his crying. After all, a man has a right to cry too.

When we find ourselves in real trouble, completely burned out, we need the help of close friends and family. We can't get along in this world without a great family and close friends.

I once read years ago of a man whose wagon got stuck in a ditch. He waited and waited until finally a friend came along and offered to help him out. They worked together for over an hour, and at last were able to get the wagon out of the mud and back on the road. The man who had been stuck in the mud was so grateful to his helper that he said, "I want you to know that if I ever come up to you and you are stuck in the mud, I'll stop and do anything I can to help you. And if I can't help you, I'll climb up on the wagon and sit beside you until help does come." Sometimes that is about all we can do for someone who is in real trouble, but merely our presence is very important to that person.

I will never forget a special, great lady who stopped by to see me. Her attitude toward life was most inspiring and impressive. She came in to see me and told me that she had just learned that she had cancer and would live but a very short time. She asked me some questions and I gave her the answers. Then, she started talking about how great each day of her life had been, how much she loved her husband, children, and all the members of her family. Then she talked about how great *each moment*, not each day, of her life had been. She was so positive about her life. Her attitude and beautiful smile were something I had never seen before in this situation. Just think, she had just been told that she had only a few short months to live. But she was such a great lady and seemed so much at peace. Then she said, "I am happy because I am still on this earth with so many people I love very much. It is not the number of years that we live that really count."

She stood up and walked over to the window in my office and asked me to join her as she was looking out into the yard filled with flowers and trees. She asked me to look at the birds playing, the puffy white clouds in the sky. She pointed out to me some things that I had never seen before, even though I look out that window every day. She really taught me how to live and enjoy live. How I wish my attitude toward each moment of my life could be just the way hers was.

Then she said, "In this magnificent world in which we live, we should never forget that if we shoot for the moon and miss we will still end up in the stars.''

Let me share with you the way a good friend has paraphrased the Optimist Creed:

I PROMISE MYSELF

I promise myself . . . to help any person that I find in need.
If by only a word . . . to make them feel they are really worth-
while.
To be so strong . . . that the troubles I find will not disturb my
peace of mind.
I will always look on the sunny side.
I will always strive for the best and do all that I can.
But, I'll praise the success of my fellowman.
I will keep so busy, I will have no time to criticize
other people.
So when I come to the end of a day, I can put my thoughts and
my work away.
I will have that feeling as I take my rest that throughout this
day, I have done my best.

Yes, I promise myself to help any person that I find in need. And I've kept that promise, but I must agree that the one person I've helped most *has really been me. You can't take care of someone else unless you also take very good care of yourself.*

Offsetting Burnout in the Thanatologic Setting: Recognition and Emphasis of "Psychosocial Successes" in Social Work Intervention

Elizabeth J. Clark

All individuals experience stress, but burnout is a distinctive type of work-related stress. In recent years, researchers have paid increasing attention to work stress and its effects on the physical and mental health of the workers. There is now a consensus that work stress can have a deleterious effect on the individual worker, on job performance, and on interpersonal relationships (Cray and Cray 1977; Farber 1983; Jayarante et al. 1986; Maslach 1983; Perlman and Hartman 1982).

Maslach, who conducted some of the pioneering research, defined burnout as "a syndrome of emotional exhaustion and cynicism that frequently occurs among individuals who do 'people work'—spend considerable time in close encounters with others under conditions of chronic tension and stress" (Maslach and Jackson 1979). There appears to be agreement regarding the symptoms of burnout—exhaustion, detachment, boredom and cynicism, impotence, a feeling of being unappreciated, paranoia, disorientation, psychosomatic complaints, depressions, and denial of feelings (Freudenberger 1980, p. 61)—but much work remains to be done in preventing and relieving the burnout syndrome.

The phenomenon of burnout originally focused on the "helping

Elizabeth J. Clark, ACSW, PhD, is Assistant Professor, Department of Health Professions, Montclair State College, Upper Montclair, NJ.

professions'' (Cherniss 1980), such as social work, and it is a sub-set of this group which this paper will address. Professionals who have been identified as particularly vulnerable to burnout are those health care providers who work in hospital settings with seriously ill patients and their families. Vachon (1979) emphasized that hospice workers are also at high risk. The major identifying characteristic of these two groups with regard to burnout is their frequent encounters with death and grief.

Numerous factors are related to the development of burnout in the thanatologic setting. These include structural factors such as inadequate support and inadequate training, pitfalls of the medical model when applied to thanatologic counseling and intervention, and lack of recognition of professional effectiveness.

STRUCTURAL FACTORS RELATED TO BURNOUT

Structural factors inadvertently contribute to the burnout syndrome. Two that are closely related are inadequate support and inadequate training.

With regard to institutional support, it is the rare program that understands the special needs of the professionals who work primarily with patients in terminal stages of illness. Responses to these needs may even take the form of "blaming the victim," that is, "you chose to work in this area, so don't ask for any special considerations." What is needed is more flexibility in scheduling, structured peer support, and increased vacation and professional days.

What is also needed is a supervisor who is sensitive to these problems and is willing to work to convince administration to make allowances for alternative scheduling and better support mechanisms. These concerns may become particularly problematic when there is only one staff person to consider, such as a designated oncology or hospice worker within a large social work department.

Inadequate training and supervision are other factors to consider when examining burnout. There are many health care professionals who are untrained or poorly trained in thanatology, and this includes supervisors and those responsible for student training. The following are two examples of poor training and inadequate supervision within the context of a caseload of terminal patients.

Example 1. A beginning pastoral counseling student expressed an interest in working on an oncology unit after completion of her hospital training program. As a result, she was immediately assigned a caseload of terminally ill cancer patients. Within the first two weeks, several of her patients died. When she complained about feeling depressed, the other students were not particularly sympathetic because she had indicated that she wished to gain experience with cancer patients, and her supervisor said she had better get used to dying patients if she ever intended to work on an oncology unit. The student eventually sought out an ancillary network in the hospital for support, and never became fully integrated into her peer group.

Example 2. A graduate social work student chose a concentration in thanatology. For her field placement, she was assigned to a medium-sized social work department within a community hospital. She was supervised by the director of the department. The other social workers were quite happy to leave the terminally ill patients to the graduate student, and she rapidly acquired a caseload composed primarily of dying patients. Yet, during her weekly supervision conference, the director refused to review or discuss the terminally ill patients because he felt it was "too depressing." The student, therefore, was denied an opportunity to learn from analysis of her intervention activities, and was also denied potentially valuable support from the director. Nor were the other social workers interested in discussing her terminally ill caseload with her. As a result, the student felt isolated and alienated from the department, and she began to question whether she had made a mistake in choosing thanatology as a specialty.

Both of these students were quickly susceptible to burnout because they lacked adequate support, and their work in thanatology was seen as less desirable than that of their co-workers who worked with less seriously ill patients.

PITFALLS OF THE MEDICAL MODEL

Just as others in the medical sphere, the social worker sees the patient's death as failure — failure of the health care system, failure of medical technology, failure of the health care team, and personal failure. Internalization of personal failure and its resulting powerlessness contribute significantly to the burnout syndrome.

Only in the last few years have we begun to study "quality of life," and many of the studies attempt to document that the quality of a terminally ill patient's life may not warrant such aggressive medical intervention as is now technologically possible.

A large literature on "death with dignity" has been developing, and the hospice movement has a program goal of helping the patient to live as "fully" as possible until death. Despite the research and the philosophy, little seems to be written about what actually constitutes "quality of life," and, as a result, it becomes difficult to know if we have succeeded in helping the terminally ill patient live "fully." In light of this, it is important to discuss the uniqueness of thanatologic counseling and the necessity of refocusing the goals for intervention with patients who are terminally ill. Particularly essential is understanding that effectiveness should be evaluated by process, not outcome, measures.

THANATOLOGIC COUNSELING INTERVENTION

Shneidman has emphasized that "working intensively with a dying person is different from almost any other human encounter" (1978, p. 206), and he identifies the different effects of psychotherapy with the dying. Foremost, it must be understood that the intervention goals are different, and that the main point is to increase the dying individual's "psychological comfort." With regard to thanatologic intervention, Shneidman contended that "the criterion of 'effectiveness' lies in this single measure" (1978, p. 212). From this perspective, it should be apparent that outcome cannot be the evaluative measure because, when working with patients who are terminally ill, by definition, the result will be the death of the patient. Instead, the evaluation measure of effectiveness must lie in the process of exchange between the professional and the patient and in the possible successes along the way. I refer to this concept as "psychosocial success," and see it as distinct from, although not always unrelated to, medical successes (or medical failures).

PSYCHOSOCIAL SUCCESSES

Psychosocial successes may be defined as those identifiable and significant events facilitated by the health care professional which contribute to the emotional well-being of the terminally ill patient and his or her family and friends. A corollary to this concept is that a psychosocial success should also have a positive effect on the health care professionals who are involved, and as a result, should be a partial antidote to burnout.

Two brief examples may help to clarify the concepts of psychosocial success.

> Example 1. Mrs. A was a 52-year-old woman diagnosed in January with melanoma of the left axilla. She underwent surgery and had follow-up radiation therapy in February and March. In August, metastasis to the lung was discovered, and she began a very aggressive course of chemotherapy. It failed to stop the spread of her disease.
>
> Mrs. A was happily married and the mother of two daughters, one aged 17 and one who would graduate from college in December. Mrs. A was close to her children and was particularly proud of her oldest daughter's academic achievements.
>
> As her disease progressed, Mrs. A realized that she was terminally ill. She maintained that her greatest desire was to live to see her daughter graduate from college.
>
> As the weeks between August and December went by, the melanoma spread through most of her left breast, and it became exceedingly painful for her to move or sit up. About mid-December, she was admitted to the hospital for pain control.
>
> It became apparent that Mrs. A would be unable to attend the graduation ceremony. Medical and nursing staff were even doubtful that she would live the few remaining days until the graduation date. However, as is so often the case, Mrs. A did

reach her goal and lived until graduation. While she could not attend the actual graduation ceremony (at a college in a nearby town), arrangements were made for her daughter to come to the hospital in her graduation gown prior to the ceremony, instant photographs were taken during the ceremony, and a small graduation party was held in Mrs. A's hospital room after her daughter had received her diploma. The nurses and social workers who had worked together to help make the plans and arrangements shared Mrs. A's and her family's happiness. When Mrs. A died 4 days later, there was sadness among the health care team, but it was somewhat tempered by the knowledge of the psychosocial success that Mrs. A did manage to participate in her daughter's graduation, and that the staff had been helpful in bringing this about. They could not prevent Mrs. A's death, but they did contribute to her emotional well-being during her final days.

Example 2. Mrs. C was a 48-year-old divorced woman who discovered a lump in her right breast. She reported it to her family physician who examined it and decided to "watch it." This "watching" continued for almost 18 months. Finally, Mrs. C's son convinced his mother that she needed to get a second opinion, and Mrs. C was directed to a surgeon. A biopsy revealed breast cancer, and further tests showed metastasis to the bone. Mrs. C spent eight months undergoing a combination of radiation therapy and chemotherapy, but the spread of the cancer continued. She also took a fall which resulted in a pathological fracture of her left ankle. Fear of further bone weakness and more fractures led to her being wheelchair bound.

Mrs. C had one exceptionally close female friend, and they had an unusual joint hobby. For 19 consecutive years, they had gone deer hunting together during the open hunting season in December. One of Mrs. C's wishes was to go deer hunting for the 20th year. While Mrs. C was scheduled to be released from the hospital directly prior to the start of hunting season, her continuing weakened condition and her inability to walk due to the ankle fracture made deer hunting appear to be an unreasonable goal. However, consultation with the friend revealed that she was more than willing to do anything possible to help make Mrs. C's desire a reality. Through combined efforts, a van was engaged for one day. The friend drove the van up into the mountains. The van had a sliding side door from which Mrs. C, seated in her wheelchair, could see into the woods and watch for deer.

They did not shoot a deer that day, but they did relive 19 years of memories of their friendship and had an opportunity to say good-by to one another. The day after the hunting trip, Mrs. C was readmitted to the hospital, and she died quietly two weeks later. During these weeks she spoke frequently about the wonderful hunting trip she had had.

Other examples of psychosocial successes with terminally ill patients are events such as returning to work one more time, being in a loved one's wedding, or taking one more trip to a favorite spot. On the surface, the idea of recounting psychosocial successes appears to be a simplistic concept. Most health care professionals can readily identify instances where they significantly helped a terminally ill patient to achieve a goal — one about which they felt especially good. Yet, few of these successes, and the roles the health care professionals played, have been documented or even recognized by others. These events have been overshadowed by the death of the patients, by the medical failure. It is the outcome, not the process, that is remembered, and it disallows the professionals the opportunity to see how effective their interventions had been. This contributes to a feeling of powerlessness to make a difference, and eventually to burnout.

APPLICATION OF SUCCESS CONCEPT IN PRACTICE AND SUPERVISION

One way to use psychosocial success to offset burnout is for the worker to accumulate a personal record of those events which contributed to the emotional well-being of terminally ill patients and their families, and which helped them to live more fully despite their terminal stage of illness. The events should be formally documented, perhaps in a log or journal format, and they must be recognized by others as effective interventions. The supervisor may want to review the worker's log during the weekly or monthly supervisory conferences. Psychosocial successes should be presented together with problems at case conferences and on psychosocial rounds. Too often we dwell on the immediate problems and crises, and neglect to recount the positive achievements.

When only failures and problems are recognized, workers begin to doubt their own usefulness and question whether or not their work has had meaning. Their powerlessness in the face of an adversary such as death is highlighted, and their effectiveness is negated. This leads quickly to burnout.

When staff morale is low, a useful tactic is to schedule a staff meeting where *only* psychosocial successes are presented, and the supervisor should insist that each person make a contribution about a successful intervention in the recent past. This will force the worker to look critically at his or her work and to take note of the positive impact he or she can and does have. Workers who see their role as ineffective tend to downplay their accomplishments and sometimes do not even recognize them. They must be given encouragement and the opportunity to emphasize their psychosocial successes, and they need to hear from peers and supervisors that they are making a difference.

CONCLUSION

Burnout is a major problem in thanatologic settings, but it is generally temporary, and it is usually reversible. Furthermore, it can be offset by sensitive supervisors who incorporate mechanisms to help staff deal more effectively with this potential problem. Most importantly, the worker must not be allowed to see death as personal failure. Instead, he or she must be encouraged to recognize the positive aspects of his or her intervention. The use of the psychosocial success concept is one approach to managing, and perhaps even preventing, the burnout syndrome.

REFERENCES

Cray, C. and M. Cray 1977. "Stress and strains within the psychiatrist's family." *American Journal of Psychoanalysis, 37*: 337-341.

Cherniss, Cary 1980. *Staff Burnout: Job Stress in the Human Services*. Beverly Hills, CA: Sage.

Farber, B.A. (Ed.) 1983. *Stress and Burnout in the Human Services Professions*. New York, NY: Pergamon.

Freudenberger, Herbert J. 1980. *Burn-out: The High Cost of Achievement*. Garden City, NY: Doubleday and Co.

Jayarante, S., Chess, W. and D. Kunkel 1986. "Burnout: Its impact on child welfare workers and their spouses." *Social Work, 31*(1): 53-59.

Maslach, C. 1983. *Burnout—The Cost of Caring*. Englewood Cliffs, NJ: Prentice-Hall.

Maslach, C. and S.E. Jackson 1979. "Burned-out cops and their families." *Psychology Today, 12*(12): 59-62.

Perlman, B. and E.A. Hartman 1982. "Burnout: Survey and future research." *Human Relations, 35*: 283-305.

Shneidman, Edwin S. 1978. "Some aspects of psychotherapy with dying patients." In C.A. Garfield (Ed.), *Psychosocial Care of the Dying Patient*. New York, NY: McGraw-Hill.

Vachon, M.L.S. 1979. "Staff stress in care of the terminally ill." *Quality Review Bulletin, 251*: 13-17.